# Artificial Intelligence in Biomedical Sciences and Healthcare

Artificial intelligence (AI) offers tremendous opportunities to transform healthcare by reducing human error, supporting medical professionals, and providing continuous patient services. With ongoing advancements, AI has demonstrated significant potential in medical imaging, such as interpreting X-rays, scans, and other diagnostics, as well as assisting in disease identification and treatment planning. Beyond clinical applications, AI is streamlining healthcare operations—from managing patient interactions and answering queries to analyzing population-level health data and predicting emerging health trends.

The book, *Artificial Intelligence in Biomedical Sciences and Healthcare*, serves as a comprehensive collection of current research on AI and its applications across diverse areas of biochemical and medical sciences. It not only presents recent advances in AI but also introduces the foundational concepts of biomedical sciences and machine learning, enabling students and professionals to better grasp these interdisciplinary fields.

Furthermore, the book addresses real-world challenges in healthcare—such as diagnostics, treatment, and disease management—and illustrate how AI-driven techniques can provide innovative solutions. This volume aims to serve as a valuable reference for students, researchers, academicians, and professionals engaged in biomedical sciences and AI.

## Advances in Bionanotechnology

**Series Editors: Ravindra Pratap Singh,** *Department of Biotechnology, Indira Gandhi National Tribal University, Anuppur, Madhya Pradesh, India,* **Jay Singh,** *Department of Chemistry, Institute of Science, Banaras Hindu University, Varanasi, Uttar Pradesh, India and* **Charles Oluwaseun Adetunji,** *Department of Microbiology, Edo State University Uzairue, Iyamho, Edo State, Nigeria*

Bionanotechnology is a multi-disciplinary field that shows immense applicability in different domains, namely chemistry, physics, material sciences, biomedical, agriculture, environment, robotics, aeronautics, energy, electronics and so forth. This book series will explore the enormous utility of bionanotechnology for biomedical, agricultural, environmental, food technology, space industry, and many other fields. It aims to highlight all the spheres of bionanotechnological applications and its safety and regulations for using biogenic nanomaterials that are a key focus of the researchers globally.

**Bionanotechnology towards Green Energy**
Innovative and Sustainable Approach
*Edited by Shubha Dwivedi and Naveen Dwivedi*

**Biotic Stress Management of Crop Plants using Nanomaterials**
*Edited by Krishna Kant Mishra and Santosh Kumar*

**Bionanotechnology for Advanced Applications**
*Edited by Ajaya Kumar Singh and Bhawana Jain*

**Nanoarchitectonics for Brain Drug Delivery**
*Edited by Anurag Kumar Singh, Vivek K. Chaturvedi and Jay Singh*

**Functional Fluorescent Materials**
Applications in Sensing, Bioimaging, and Optoelectronics
*Edited by Vivek Mishra, Syed Sibtay Razi and Ajit Kumar*

**Nanotherapeutics for Inflammatory Arthritis**
Design, Diagnosis, and Treatment
*Edited by Vivek Mishra, Ramendrapati Pandey, Anjali Priyadarshini, Chung-Ming Chang and Elcio Leal*

**Piezoelectric as Smart Biomaterials for Cardiovascular Tissue Regeneration**
*Edited by Rakesh Bhaskar, Santosh Kumar and Mukesh Kumar Gupta*

**Artificial Intelligence in Biomedical Sciences and Healthcare**
*Edited by Imran Khan and Santosh Kumar*

For more information about this series, please visit: www.routledge.com/Advances-in-Bionanotechnology/book-series/CRCBIONAN

# Artificial Intelligence in Biomedical Sciences and Healthcare

Edited by
Imran Khan
and Santosh Kumar

CRC Press
Taylor & Francis Group
Boca Raton London New York

CRC Press is an imprint of the
Taylor & Francis Group, an **informa** business

Designed cover image: Shutterstock

First edition published 2026
by CRC Press
2385 NW Executive Center Drive, Suite 320, Boca Raton FL 33431

and by CRC Press
4 Park Square, Milton Park, Abingdon, Oxon, OX14 4RN

*CRC Press is an imprint of Taylor & Francis Group, LLC*



ISBN: 9781032865744 (hbk)
ISBN: 9781041243991 (pbk)
ISBN: 9781003741770 (ebk)

DOI: 10.1201/9781003741770

Typeset in Sabon
by Deanta Global Publishing Services, Chennai, India

# Contents

*Preface* vii
*Editor biographies* ix
*List of contributors* x

1 Role of artificial intelligence in healthcare and biomedical science 1
IMRAN KHAN, BRAJESH KUMAR KHARE, ASAD MALIK, AND SANTOSH KUMAR

2 Applications of artificial intelligence in healthcare 26
RASHMI RAMESHWARI, NAINA SONI, DEVENDRA KUMAR VERMA, AND SANTOSH KUMAR

3 Artificial intelligence in the treatment and diagnosis of infectious diseases 51
MOHMMAD YOUNUS WANI

4 The role of artificial intelligence in diabetes: A review of recent advances 67
MRIDUL SHARMA, GAURAV KUMAR, SANTOSH KUMAR, SHALINEE SINGH, PREM ANURAG, AND IMRAN KHAN

5 Artificial intelligence in gynecology 81
SHALINEE SINGH, SANTOSH KUMAR, SUNDARARAJAN V. MADIHALLY, AND IMRAN KHAN

6 Role of AI in gastroenterology: Prevention, diagnostics, and treatment 99
IMRAN KHAN, BRAJESH KUMAR KHARE, MOHAMMAD SHOAIB KHAN, AND SANTOSH KUMAR

7 Artificial intelligence in drug delivery 116

IRA SINGH, SANTOSH KUMAR, JOONSEOK KOH, AND ABILIO J.F.N. SOBRAL

8 Artificial intelligence in genomics 150

RASHMI RAMESHWARI, ADHIKARKA SYAMA, SRINIVASAN RAMACHANDRAN, DEVENDRA KUMAR VERMA, AND SANTOSH KUMAR

9 Trends and challenges in the field of medical sciences using AI 167

RASHMI RAMESHWARI, SONIA KAUSHIK, SRINIVASAN RAMACHANDRAN, DEVENDRA KUMAR VERMA, AND SANTOSH KUMAR

10 A survey of clinical decision support systems 188

VINAYAK GUPTA, YAJNASENI DASH, DINESH KUMAR, NAWEEN KUMAR, AND SUDHIR C. SARANGI

*Index* 199

# Preface

Artificial intelligence (AI) provides opportunities to help reduce human error, assist medical professionals and staff, and provide patient services 24/7. As AI tools continue to develop, there is potential to use AI even more in reading medical images such as X-rays and scans, diagnosing medical problems, and creating treatment plans. AI applications will continue to help streamline various tasks, from answering phones to analyzing population health trends (and, likely, applications yet to be considered). For instance, future AI tools may automate or augment more of the work of clinicians and staff members. This will free up humans to spend more time on more effective and compassionate face-to-face professional care.

The book *Artificial Intelligence in Biomedical Sciences and Healthcare* is an outstanding collection of current research on artificial intelligence with its applications in various domains of Biochemical and Medical Sciences. It also provides an overview of selected advances that have taken place in the field of AI. Moreover, this book introduces the basic concepts of Biomedical Sciences and Machine Learning to help students and professionals to better understand these fields. In addition, it helps them understand and address day-to-day problems related to human health, diagnostics, and treatments and how AI overcomes these challenges by using different techniques. This book will serve as a reference book for professionals, students, scientists, researchers, and academicians in this subject area. We hope that readers will find it beneficial to their future research and teaching endeavors.

The book *Artificial Intelligence in Biomedical Sciences and Healthcare* will attract a wide range of readers from various research fields, as this book provides the fundamental aspects of Biochemical and Biomedical Sciences and AI with their applications. Additionally, this book provides a platform for the scientific community, working on various aspects of artificial intelligence, machine learning, deep learning etc., to share new advancements. Our ambition is that the book offers highlights of recent research developments to experienced researchers and introduces this fascinating research field to beginners. Chapter 1 deals with artificial intelligence and biomedical sciences, including research trends in both domains and open research areas. Chapter 2 provides insights into different applications of artificial intelligence in healthcare. Chapter 3 deals with artificial intelligence in the treatment and diagnosis of infectious diseases. Chapter 4 deals with the role of artificial intelligence in diabetes: a review of recent advances. Chapter 5 deals with recent progress in the field of gynecology with the advances in AI. Chapter 6 deals with the role of AI in gastroenterology: prevention, diagnostics, and treatment. Chapter 7 deals with artificial intelligence in drug delivery. Chapter 8 deals with artificial intelligence in genomics. Chapter 9 deals with the trends and challenges in the field of medical sciences using AI. Chapter 10 deals with a survey of clinical decision support systems.

# Editor biographies

**Imran Khan** is currently working as Assistant Professor at the Department of Computer Science and Engineering, Harcourt Butler Technical University, Kanpur, India. He completed his PhD from Jamia Millia Islamia, New Delhi, India. He did his master's in computer applications from Aligarh Muslim University, Aligarh, India. He has experience in both industries and teaching. He worked as Senior Data Scientist at Crysp Analytics, Noida, India. Also, he worked as Assistant Professor at BVICAM, New Delhi. He published more than 20 research papers in various journals and conferences. His area of research is Artificial Intelligence, Machine Learning, Deep Learning and Data Science.

**Santosh Kumar** is currently working as Associate Professor and Head of the Department of Chemistry, Harcourt Butler Technical University, Kanpur, India. He also served as Research Professor in the Department of Organic and Nano System Engineering, Division of Chemical Engineering, Konkuk University, Seoul, South Korea. Dr Kumar received his BSc and MSc in chemistry and DPhil in organic chemistry from the University of Allahabad, India. He worked as Research Associate (CSIR) at the Department of Chemistry, Motilal Nehru National Institute of Technology, Allahabad, India. He was awarded the CAS-TWAS Postdoctoral fellowship in 2008 and worked at the Changchun Institute of Applied Chemistry, Chinese Academy of Sciences, Changchun, China. Later, he joined as a KU Brain Pool Professor and researcher at Konkuk University, Seoul, South Korea (2010–2013). He was awarded the FCT Postdoctoral Fellowship 2012 and worked at the Chemistry Centre, University of Coimbra, Coimbra, Portugal (2013–2017). During his career, Dr Kumar has published more than 121 research papers, edited 6 books and 28 book chapters, and attended and participated in local and international workshops and conferences. He also served as a member of different organizing committees and an editorial board member and a reviewer for a number of scientific journals. His current research interest involves source apportionment of chemical modification, optical and biological properties of chitosan biopolymer for biomedical applications, hydrogels, aerogels, nanomaterials, porous organic polymers and drug and gene delivery.

# Contributors

**Anurag, Prem**
School of Basic and Applied Sciences
Galgotias University
Greater Noida, India

**Dash, Yajnaseni**
School of Artificial Intelligence
Bennett University
Greater Noida, India

**Gupta, Vinayak**
School of Computer Science Engineering and Technology
Bennett University
Greater Noida, India

**Kaushik, Sonia**
Department of Biotechnology
School of Engineering and Technology
Manav Rachna International Institute of Research and Studies
Faridabad, India

**Khare, Brajesh Kumar**
Department of Computer Science and Engineering
Harcourt Butler Technical University
Kanpur, India

**Khan, Imran**
Department of Computer Science and Engineering
Harcourt Butler Technical University
Kanpur, India

**Koh, Joonseok**
Department of Materials Science and Engineering
Konkuk University
Seoul, South Korea

**Kumar, Dinesh**
School of Artificial Intelligence
Bennett University
Greater Noida, India

**Kumar, Gaurav**
Department of Biotechnology and Bioengineering
School of Biosciences and Technology
Galgotias University
Greater Noida, India

**Kumar, Naween**
School of Computer Science Engineering and Technology
Bennett University
Greater Noida, India

**Kumar, Santosh**
Department of Chemistry
Harcourt Butler Technical University
Kanpur, India

**Madihally, Sundararajan V.**
Oklahoma State University
Stillwater, OK

**Malik, Asad**
School of Information Technology
Monash University
Malaysia

**Ramachandran, Srinivasan**
Research Development Cell
Manav Rachna International Institute of Research and Studies
Faridabad, India

**Rameshwari, Rashmi**
Department of Biotechnology
School of Engineering and Technology
Manav Rachna International Institute of Research and Studies
Faridabad, India

**Sarangi, Sudhir C.**
Department of Pharmacology
AIIMS
New Delhi, India

**Sharma, Mridul**
Department of Biomedical Sciences
Galgotias University
Greater Noida, India

**Shoaib, Mohammad Khan**
Department of Management and Social Sciences
Amity University
Tashkent, Uzbekistan

**Soni, Naina**
Department of Biotechnology
School of Engineering and Technology
Manav Rachna International Institute of Research and Studies
Faridabad, India

**Singh, Ira**
Department of Chemistry
School of Basic and Applied Sciences
Harcourt Butler Technical University
Kanpur, India

**Singh, Shalinee**
Department of Chemistry
Harcourt Butler Technical University
Kanpur, India

**Sobral, Abilio J.F.N.**
Department of Chemistry
University of Coimbra
Coimbra, Portugal

**Syama, Adhikarka**
Pitch Foundation
Madurai, India

**Verma, Devendra Kumar**
Department of Chemistry
Raja Mahendra Pratap Singh State University
Aligarh, India

**Wani, Mohmmad Younus**
Department of Chemistry
College of Science
University of Jeddah
Jeddah, Saudi Arabia

Chapter 1

# Role of artificial intelligence in healthcare and biomedical science

*Imran Khan, Brajesh Kumar Khare, Asad Malik, and Santosh Kumar*

## 1.1 INTRODUCTION

In today's world, technology is transforming healthcare, with one of the most exciting developments being artificial intelligence (AI), a super-smart program that learns from data and makes decisions independently [1]. This study is all about exploring how AI is being used in healthcare to make things better for patients and doctors alike. Imagine going to the doctor and getting a diagnosis faster and more accurately than ever before—that's what AI can do. It helps doctors analyze medical images, like X-rays and magnetic resonance imaging (MRI), to spot diseases such as cancer sooner. Studies, such as the one by Esteva et al. [2], show that AI can even match the expertise of dermatologists in spotting skin cancer from images. But AI isn't just about images. It also helps doctors make decisions about treatments. For example, researchers like Rajkomar et al. [3] have shown how AI can analyze vast amounts of patient records to suggest the best treatments based on what worked for similar patients in the past. This kind of personalized medicine could lead to faster recoveries and fewer side effects for patients. And it doesn't stop there. AI is also playing a significant role in drug discovery. By crunching data and running simulations, scientists can use AI to speed up the process of discovering and testing new drugs. This means potentially life-saving treatments could reach patients much faster [4]. AI isn't just for doctors and scientists, though. It's also helping with the day-to-day tasks of running a hospital or clinic. By automating tasks like scheduling appointments and managing supplies, AI frees up time for healthcare workers to focus more on patient care. However, as exciting as all this is, there are also some important considerations. AI raises questions about privacy, fairness, and ensuring that the technology is used safely and ethically. We need to make sure that as AI becomes more common in healthcare, it benefits everyone and does not cause harm.

Before 2010, the focus of healthcare technology was on developing medical products that supported traditional, evidence-based care. These innovations aimed at improving patient outcomes based on historical data and well-established medical practices. However, after 2010, there was a shift

DOI: 10.1201/9781003741770-1

in focus toward creating real-time medical platforms that enabled more dynamic and outcome-oriented care. This change was driven by the need to address healthcare challenges more efficiently and provide better, faster solutions to patients.

By 2020, the healthcare industry began adopting more advanced and intelligent technologies to deliver evidence- and outcome-based care. The emphasis shifted toward collaborative and preventive care, which focuses on preventing diseases and working together across different medical disciplines. Technologies like robotics, virtual reality, augmented reality, and artificial intelligence have played a major role in achieving these goals. These tools not only enhance patient care but also make healthcare systems smarter and more efficient. A recent survey of life science executives revealed that 69% of companies in the field have already implemented or piloted AI in their solutions, while 22% are in the process of evaluating or planning to use AI. This shows the growing trust and interest in AI technologies across the healthcare sector. Moreover, the economic benefits are significant. AI is now being applied in many areas of healthcare, transforming the way care is delivered. Some key applications include surgery, where AI assists in precision tasks; nursing assistance, where AI supports patient care; and medical consultation, where AI aids in providing accurate recommendations. It is also improving administrative tasks and workflows, treatment planning, cybersecurity, and clinical trials. Other areas, like health monitoring, medication management, and preliminary diagnosis, are also benefiting from AI, making healthcare systems more reliable and patient-centric. These advancements demonstrate the immense potential of AI to revolutionize healthcare in the coming years.

AI has numerous applications in healthcare and biomedical science, with many researchers contributing to these areas. This chapter is organized to examine research in these fields. The structure is as follows: Section 1.2 covers healthcare research, including topics like clinical research, basic science research, and health services research. Section 1.3 discusses biomedical science. Section 1.4 explains artificial intelligence. Section 1.5 explores the clinical applications of AI in healthcare. Section 1.6 highlights the challenges of AI in healthcare and biomedical science. Section 1.7 examines the future potential of AI in these fields. Finally, Section 1.8 presents the conclusions.

## 1.2 HEALTHCARE RESEARCH

Healthcare research encompasses a vast and diverse array of scientific inquiries aimed at understanding, improving, and innovating various aspects of healthcare delivery, patient care, disease prevention, and treatment. It encompasses a wide range of disciplines, methodologies, and focus areas, driven by the common goal of advancing medical knowledge and improving health outcomes. Here's a detailed exploration of healthcare research.

### 1.2.1 Clinical research

Clinical research involves studying health and disease in humans, typically through observational studies, clinical trials, and epidemiological investigations. Clinical trials evaluate the safety and efficacy of medical treatments, drugs, devices, or interventions in human subjects. Observational studies explore relationships between risk factors, diseases, and health outcomes, while epidemiological research investigates patterns and determinants of disease occurrence and distribution within populations.

### 1.2.2 Applied research

Applied research serves as a crucial link between fundamental scientific discoveries and their application in clinical settings, transforming scientific knowledge into practical advancements in patient care. It involves multidisciplinary collaborations among scientists, clinicians, and industry partners to develop novel therapies, diagnostics, and medical technologies. Translational research encompasses various stages, including bench-to-bedside translation (from laboratory discoveries to clinical trials) and bedside-to-community translation (from clinical practice to population health interventions).

### 1.2.3 Fundamental research

Fundamental research, also known as basic science or preclinical research, investigates fundamental biological mechanisms underlying health and disease. It involves studying biological processes, molecular pathways, cellular interactions, and genetic factors using laboratory-based experiments, animal models, and computational simulations. Basic science research provides foundational knowledge that informs the development of new diagnostics, treatments, and preventive strategies.

### 1.2.4 Community health research

Community health research aims to enhance and safeguard the well-being of populations by implementing strategies for disease prevention, health promotion, and policy-based interventions in patient care. It encompasses epidemiological studies, health behavior research, environmental health investigations, health disparities research, and health services research. Public health researchers aim to identify risk factors, develop interventions, and implement policies to improve population health outcomes and reduce health inequities.

### 1.2.5 Medical services research

Medical services research focuses on studying the structure, provision, and use of medical services to enhance their quality, accessibility, and overall efficiency. It involves studying healthcare delivery systems, healthcare financing, healthcare disparities, patient outcomes, and healthcare policy interventions. Health services researchers employ quantitative and qualitative methods, including health economics, health informatics, and operations research, to evaluate healthcare delivery models, healthcare technologies, and healthcare interventions.

### 1.2.6 Biomedical engineering and technology research

Biomedical engineering and technology research focuses on developing innovative medical devices, diagnostics, imaging technologies, and therapeutic modalities to improve patient care and clinical outcomes. It encompasses disciplines such as biomedical engineering, bioinformatics, medical imaging, telemedicine, and wearable health technologies. Biomedical engineers collaborate with clinicians, scientists, and industry partners to design, prototype, and validate new healthcare technologies for clinical use.

### 1.2.7 Global health research

Global health research addresses health challenges that transcend national boundaries, with a focus on improving health equity, reducing health disparities, and addressing global health threats. It emphasizes the study of both infectious and non-communicable diseases, the advancement of maternal and child health, and the strengthening of healthcare systems in areas with limited resources. Global health researchers collaborate across disciplines and regions to develop contextually appropriate interventions and strategies for improving health outcomes worldwide.

### 1.2.8 Health policy and health economics research

Health policy and health economics research examine the impact of healthcare policies, regulations, and financing mechanisms on health outcomes, healthcare access, and healthcare costs. It involves evaluating the effectiveness of healthcare interventions, analyzing healthcare expenditure trends, and assessing the economic value of healthcare innovations. Health policy researchers provide evidence-based recommendations to policymakers to inform healthcare policy decisions and improve health system performance.

## 1.3 BIOMEDICAL SCIENCE

Biomedical science explores the mechanisms behind the functioning of the human body and the development of diseases, using biology, medicine, and advanced technologies to improve healthcare. This field explores everything from the smallest molecules in the body, such as DNA and proteins, to the coordinated function of entire systems, such as the heart and immune system, which work together to maintain health. The main goal is to use this knowledge to develop new treatments, medicines, and technologies for diagnosing and curing diseases. One key area is genetics, where scientists study how our genes influence health. For example, understanding genetic mutations has helped predict diseases like cancer, and the emergence of personalized medicine has paved the way for treatments specifically designed to suit an individual's genetic profile [5]. This approach is transforming healthcare by allowing doctors to target treatments more effectively.

Biomedical science is also at the forefront of fighting diseases through drug discovery and vaccine development. A great example is the rapid development of COVID-19 vaccines. Researchers combined traditional biology with modern tools, like artificial intelligence (AI), to speed up the process of identifying effective vaccines [6]. AI helped analyze large datasets of genetic information and predict how the virus would behave, making it possible to create vaccines in record time.

In regenerative medicine, biomedical scientists use stem cells to repair or replace damaged tissues. For instance, stem cell therapy holds significant potential in addressing spinal cord injuries, cardiac conditions, and vision loss. Additionally, breakthroughs in 3D printing technology are being utilized to develop customized artificial organs and implants designed specifically for individual patients [7].

Another critical area is understanding infectious diseases, like malaria or tuberculosis, and developing tools to diagnose and treat them. Using genomic sequencing and bioinformatics, researchers can track disease outbreaks and design targeted treatments, which is essential for global health.

Despite these advances, biomedical science faces challenges. Ethical questions arise when using technologies like Clustered Regularly Interspaced Short Palindromic Repeats (CRISPR) to edit genes, particularly when editing human embryos [8]. Data privacy is another concern, especially as the collection of genetic data continues to increase. Additionally, ensuring that these technologies are accessible and affordable remains a significant hurdle.

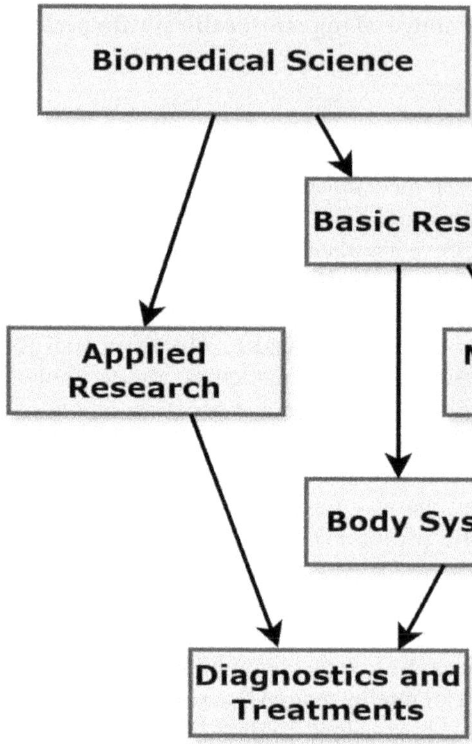


*Figure 1.1* Biomedical science

The fusion of biomedical science with cutting-edge technologies such as AI, robotics, and big data is set to redefine healthcare. These breakthroughs promise transformative advancements in disease treatment and a deeper comprehension of life, fostering global health and well-being.

Figure 1.1 shows the fundamental pathway of biomedical science, while Table 1.1 summarizes key aspects of biomedical science.

## 1.4 ARTIFICIAL INTELLIGENCE

Computers are now able to think and act like humans with the help of AI technologies. These intelligent machines can learn, solve problems, and make decisions in ways similar to humans. They analyze large amounts of data to find patterns and gain understanding, which helps them make smart choices. Scientists have developed various types of AI that can recognize human speech, process images, control robots, and improve skills through practice.

*Table 1.1* Key aspects of biomedical science

| *Aspect* | *Description* | *Techniques used* | *Applications* | *Challenges* | *Future prospects* |
|---|---|---|---|---|---|
| Research areas | Investigates biological processes and mechanisms underlying health and disease | Microscopy, PCR, gel electrophoresis | Disease pathology, cellular biology | Data complexity, funding constraints | Advanced genomic techniques, personalized medicine |
| Genomics and proteomics | Studies genes and proteins to understand their functions and interactions | Sequencing, mass spectrometry | Genetic disorder research, drug target identification | Ethical issues, data security | Integration with CRISPR, proteomics advancements |
| Cell and molecular biology | Examines cellular structures, functions, and molecular interactions | Cell culture, flow cytometry | Cancer research, stem cell therapy | Experimental complexity, reproducibility | Organoid models, single-cell analysis |
| Biomedical imaging | Utilizes imaging technologies to visualize biological tissues and structures | MRI, CT, PET, ultrasound | Diagnostic imaging, surgical planning | Image resolution, interpretation accuracy | AI-enhanced imaging, 3D imaging techniques |
| Pharmacology | Explores drug interactions, efficacy, and safety | Drug screening, in vivo models | Drug development, toxicology studies | Side effects, patient variability | Targeted drug delivery, nanomedicine |
| Immunology | Studies the immune system and its responses | ELISA, western blotting, cytokine assays | Vaccine development, autoimmune research | Autoimmunity, pathogen resistance | Immunotherapy, personalized vaccines |
| Neuroscience | Investigates the nervous system, brain functions, and neurological disorders | Electrophysiology, brain imaging | Neurodegenerative disease research, brain–machine interface | Complexity of neural networks, ethical concerns | Neuroprosthetics, advanced neural imaging techniques |
| Bioinformatics | Applies computational tools to analyze biological data | Data mining, machine learning | Genomic data analysis, protein structure prediction | Data overload, integration challenges | AI-driven analysis, big data integration |
| Ethical considerations | Addresses the ethical implications and standards in biomedical research | Ethical reviews, consent procedures | Human subject research, clinical trials | Privacy concerns, informed consent | Global ethical standards, enhanced transparency |

Machine learning, a branch of artificial intelligence, involves designing systems that learn from data and enhance their performance automatically, without requiring manual programming. It includes various approaches, such as supervised learning, where systems are trained with labeled data; unsupervised learning, where they uncover hidden patterns in data; and reinforcement learning, where they enhance their performance through trial and error. These methods allow machines to make accurate predictions, recognize trends, and tackle complex problems. Natural language processing (NLP) allows machines to comprehend, analyze, and produce human language. This technology powers numerous everyday applications, including language translation services, virtual assistants, chatbots, and sentiment analysis tools, improving how machines interact with humans.

Computer vision, an essential field of artificial intelligence, enables machines to understand and process visual information such as images and videos. This technology is used in tasks like recognizing objects, classifying images, detecting faces, and analyzing video feeds. Applications of computer vision include security systems, autonomous vehicles, medical imaging, and even social media filters. Robotics integrates artificial intelligence with mechanical engineering to create advanced machines capable of executing physical tasks. Robots powered by AI can work in real-world environments, such as factories, hospitals, and even outer space. Examples include autonomous vehicles, robotic surgery systems, and warehouse robots. AI has become an essential tool in many industries. In healthcare, AI is transforming the way doctors diagnose and treat diseases. Artificial intelligence (AI) holds immense potential to transform multiple industries. In healthcare, AI aids in the early identification of diseases, including cancer, by analyzing medical imaging, such as X-rays and MRIs, with remarkable accuracy. Moreover, AI can create personalized treatment strategies by evaluating a patient's genetic information and medical history. In the financial industry, AI is instrumental in detecting fraudulent activities, streamlining workflows, and improving the efficiency of decision-making processes. In the transportation sector, AI plays a crucial role in advancing self-driving vehicles and improving traffic flow management. Additionally, in retail, AI improves customer satisfaction by offering tailored suggestions and optimizing inventory management. However, despite its many benefits, AI also presents several challenges. Key concerns include data privacy, as AI relies on large amounts of personal data; job displacement, as automation replaces certain types of work; and fairness, as biases in AI systems can lead to unfair decisions. It is important to address these issues responsibly to ensure that AI is used ethically and effectively.

Overall, AI has the potential to improve lives, drive innovation, and solve many problems across different fields. As technology continues to advance, it is important to balance its development with thoughtful planning and

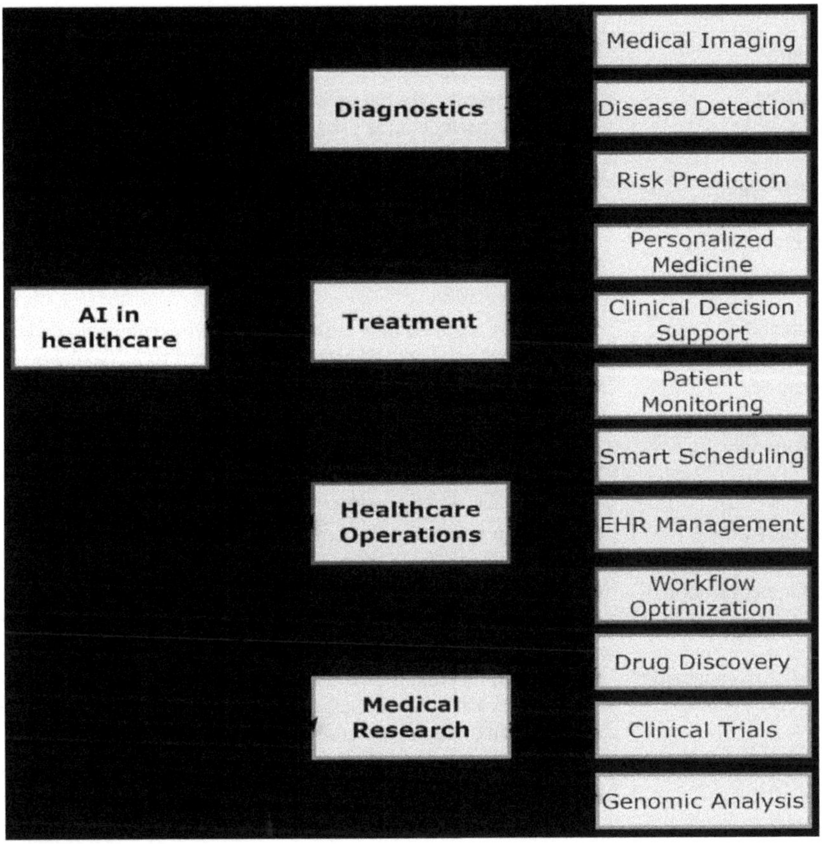


*Figure 1.2* AI in healthcare

careful handling of its challenges. Figure 1.2 illustrates the major clinical applications of AI in healthcare. Table 1.2 describes the key features of artificial intelligence.

## 1.5 CLINICAL APPLICATIONS OF AI IN HEALTHCARE

Artificial intelligence is transforming healthcare by providing new solutions in different areas, with the goal of improving patient care, making diagnoses more accurate, improving treatment plans, and reducing administrative work. Table 1.3 presents an overview of various applications of AI in healthcare, highlighting the key areas where AI is significantly transforming the healthcare industry.

*Table 1.2* Features of artificial intelligence

| *Feature* | *Description* |
|---|---|
| Learning | AI systems have the ability to analyze data and enhance their performance progressively using methods such as machine learning. |
| Reasoning | AI can use logical rules to make decisions or solve problems, often mimicking human thought processes. |
| Problem-solving | AI algorithms can analyze complex problems and generate solutions or recommendations based on available information. |
| Adaptability | AI can adapt to new situations or environments and adjust its behavior accordingly, often referred to as flexibility. |
| Creativity | Some AI systems are capable of generating novel ideas, designs, or solutions, although this feature is still evolving. |
| Autonomy | AI systems have the ability to function autonomously, making decisions and performing actions on their own in specific situations, like with self-driving cars. |
| Interaction | AI can interact with humans or other systems through interfaces like voice assistants, chatbots, or virtual agents. |
| Self-improvement | AI systems can iteratively improve their performance through feedback mechanisms, continuously refining their algorithms or models. |
| Predictive capabilities | AI can forecast future outcomes or trends based on historical data and patterns, enabling applications like predictive analytics and forecasting. |
| Perception | AI systems can perceive and interpret sensory inputs such as images, sounds, and text, through techniques like computer vision and natural language processing. |

### 1.5.1 Medical imaging and diagnostics

The field of medical imaging and diagnostics is undergoing a transformation due to the integration of AI, which significantly enhances the precision, speed, and efficiency of these processes. AI-powered algorithms are highly effective in interpreting complex medical images like X-rays, computed tomography (CT) scans, MRIs, and mammograms. These algorithms can identify patterns and anomalies that might be difficult for humans to detect at first glance. One of the most important advantages of AI in this context is its ability to spot early signs of diseases, enabling timely interventions and better outcomes for patients. AI-powered systems assist radiologists and healthcare professionals by providing precise and consistent interpretations of medical images, contributing to more reliable diagnoses and treatment strategies. These systems can effectively identify abnormalities, including tumors, fractures, and lesions, and offer quantitative data for disease assessment and progression monitoring. Additionally, AI

*Table 1.3* AI in healthcare

| *Application* | *Description* |
|---|---|
| Medical imaging and diagnostics | AI processes medical images, such as X-rays and MRI scans, to support radiologists in identifying abnormalities, tumors, fractures, and other medical conditions, thereby improving diagnostic precision. |
| Drug discovery | AI facilitates the identification of promising drug candidates, evaluates their potential effectiveness, and models drug interactions, significantly accelerating the drug discovery process. |
| Personalized treatment | AI algorithms assess patient data to tailor treatment strategies, taking into account variables such as genetic makeup, medical background, and lifestyle choices. |
| Virtual health assistants and telemedicine | AI-driven virtual assistants and chatbots offer tailored healthcare guidance, help in evaluating symptoms, and support remote monitoring, enhancing telemedicine services and online consultations. |
| Precision medicine and genomics | AI examines genomic data to uncover genetic differences, biomarkers, and predispositions to diseases, allowing for the development of personalized medicine strategies based on each patient's unique genetic makeup. |
| Robotic surgery and assistance | AI-powered surgical robots aid surgeons in conducting minimally invasive surgeries with improved accuracy and control, leading to better surgical results and faster patient recovery. |
| Healthcare operations and administration | AI streamlines administrative processes like scheduling appointments, handling billing, and performing medical coding, enhancing resource management, and boosting operational productivity. |
| Healthcare fraud detection and security | AI algorithms examine healthcare data to identify fraudulent activities, billing mistakes, and breaches of compliance, helping maintain regulatory standards and safeguard patient information. |

streamlines repetitive tasks like image segmentation and feature extraction, thereby reducing radiologists' workload and allowing them to concentrate on complex cases. AI-based diagnostic tools also integrate seamlessly with electronic health records and clinical decision-making systems, offering actionable insights and personalized recommendations based on patient information and imaging results. By improving diagnostic accuracy and efficiency, AI has the potential to enhance patient care, lower healthcare costs, and optimize healthcare services. A comprehensive summary of AI applications in medical imaging, including their benefits, limitations, and use cases, is presented in Table 1.4.

Advancements in medical imaging have been significantly enhanced by the integration of AI, particularly through deep learning (DL) methods.

*Table 1.4* AI applications in medical imaging

| *Application* | *Description* | *Benefits* | *Challenges* |
|---|---|---|---|
| Detection of abnormalities | AI examines medical images, such as X-rays and MRI scans, to identify irregularities like tumors, fractures, or lesions, supporting early detection and assisting in treatment planning. | Early detection leads to timely intervention and improved patient outcomes. | Interpretability of AI algorithms, potential false positives/negatives. |
| Image segmentation | AI automates the process of segmenting anatomical structures or regions of interest in medical images, facilitating quantitative analysis and visualization. | Accurate segmentation enables precise measurement and assessment of disease progression. | Variability in image quality, complex anatomical structures. |
| Feature extraction | AI algorithms extract relevant features or patterns from medical images, helping identify diagnostic biomarkers and distinguish between different tissue types. | Enhanced feature extraction aids in identifying subtle changes indicative of disease. | Robustness to image artifacts, generalization across diverse datasets. |
| Quantitative analysis | AI provides quantitative measurements and assessments of medical images, such as tumor volume, tissue density, or perfusion parameters, aiding in disease staging and monitoring. | Objective quantification enhances diagnostic accuracy and treatment planning. | Standardization of measurement protocols, validation against clinical gold standards. |
| Differential diagnosis | AI assists in differential diagnosis by analyzing medical images and comparing them with reference databases or clinical guidelines, aiding in accurate disease classification. | Accurate differentiation between similar conditions improves diagnostic confidence. | Incorporating clinical context, addressing rare or complex cases. |
| Personalized treatment planning | AI assists in customizing treatment strategies by analyzing individual patient traits and disease information derived from medical images, thereby enhancing therapeutic results and reducing side effects. | Personalized treatment improves patient outcomes and reduces adverse effects. | Integration with patient data, validation in clinical trials. |

(*Continued*)

*Table 1.4* (Continued) AI applications in medical imaging

| *Application* | *Description* | *Benefits* | *Challenges* |
|---|---|---|---|
| Automation of routine tasks | AI automates repetitive tasks in medical imaging workflows, such as image preprocessing, quality control, and report generation, streamlining radiologists' workflow and reducing workload. | Increased efficiency and productivity allow radiologists to focus on complex cases. | Integration with existing systems, user acceptance, and trust. |
| Clinical decision support | AI provides decision support to radiologists and clinicians by analyzing medical images and patient data, offering insights, recommendations, and alerts based on evidence-based guidelines. | Decision support tools enhance diagnostic accuracy and adherence to best practices. | Integration with clinical workflows, ensuring real-time feedback and relevance. |

Various studies have applied AI models, such as convolutional neural networks (CNNs) and transfer learning strategies, to enhance the accuracy, speed, and reliability of diagnosing and predicting diseases. The contributions of various researchers in progressing medical imaging technologies, with an emphasis on detecting and classifying diseases, are discussed in Table 1.5.

### 1.5.2 AI in drug discovery

Artificial intelligence can transform the drug discovery process by making it faster, more accurate, and more efficient. Machine learning is widely used in computer-based drug discovery [19, 20]. Deep learning techniques, including artificial neural networks (ANNs) with several hidden layers, have recently attracted considerable attention. This is mainly because they can automatically identify features from input data and capture intricate nonlinear dependencies between inputs and outputs [21]. These capabilities of deep learning offer significant improvements over conventional machine learning methods, which usually rely on manually crafted molecular descriptors [22]. Drug discovery has recently experienced a surge of interest in deep learning [23], resulting in a rapid development of new modeling approaches and applications [24, 25].

Table 1.6 presents a list of AI tools and models that play an important role in drug discovery. These models help predict the structure of proteins, find out how drugs interact with targets, predict the toxicity of chemicals, and screen compounds virtually. Each model is briefly described, focusing

*Table 1.5* Contributions of researchers in medical imaging

| *References* | *Disease* | *Imaging data* | *Patient* | *Method used* | *Description* |
|---|---|---|---|---|---|
| Lo et al. [9] | Lung cancer | X-ray | 55 | 2-layer CNN | First ever used CNN got medical image analysis |
| Ronneberger et al. [10] | cells | Electron and optical microscopy | 30/35 | U-NET | Exceptional segmentation performance with limited data |
| Dou et al. [11] | Cerebral microbleeds | MRI | 320 | 3D CNN | Detect candidate microbleeds to reduce false positives |
| Yu et al. [12] | Melanoma | Dermoscop ic images | 1250 images | Fully convolutional residual network | Binary melanoma classification |
| Lao et al. [13] | Glioblastoma Multiforme(GBM) | MRI | 112 | Transfer learning | Survical prognostic signature for patients with GBM |
| Kamnitsas et al. [14] | Traumatic brain injury (TBI), Low-grade glioma (LGG)/GBM, stroke | MRI | 61/110/ ISLES-SISS data | CNN with 11 layers, integrated with a fully connected CRF | Achieving exceptional segmentation outcomes for traumatic brain injuries (TBIs), brain tumors, and ischemic strokes |
| Zhu et al. [15] | Breast cancer | DCE-MRI | 270 | Transfer learning | Differentiate between luminal and other breast cancer types |
| Chartsias et al. [16] | Cardiovascular | MRI | 100 | Various networks | Partitioning of the cardiac structure |
| Mckinney et al. [17] | Breast cancer | X-ray | 25,856 cases | Ensemble and transfer learning | Diagnosis of breast cancer |
| Hekler et al. [18] | Melanoma | H&E tissue imaging | 695 | Transfer learning | Binary melanoma classification |

*Table 1.6* AI in drug discovery

| *References* | *Description* |
|---|---|
| AlphaFold2 [26] | A deep learning model used to predict the structure of proteins based on their amino acid sequences. |
| DeepChem [27] | A specialized deep learning framework designed to advance drug discovery and computational chemistry processes. |
| DeepBind [28] | A software tool designed to assess the interaction between proteins and DNA/RNA molecules. |
| DeepBar [29] | A technique for swiftly and precisely estimating the binding free energy. |
| DeepScreening [30] | A deep learning-driven web server for performing virtual screening of chemical compounds. |
| DeepScreen [31] | Efficient identification of drug interactions with target proteins. |
| DeepConv-DTI [32] | A CNN-based model is developed to forecast the interactions between drugs and their molecular targets. |
| DeepPurpose [33] | A deep learning model for predicting drug–target relationships, drug interactions, protein connections, and protein functions. |
| DeepTox [34] | A neural network-based system developed to predict the toxicity levels of chemical substances. |
| AtomNet [35] | An advanced convolutional neural network model developed to predict bioactivity in various biological systems. |
| PathDSP [36] | A deep learning approach to forecast the responsiveness of cancer cell lines to various drugs. |
| Chemical VAE [37] | A framework utilizing autoencoders to create novel molecular structures. |
| TorchDrug [38] | A versatile framework built on PyTorch, tailored for developing models in drug discovery. |

on how deep learning techniques like CNNs and autoencoders are used. These tools make the drug discovery process faster, more accurate, and help in developing new medicines more efficiently.

### 1.5.3 AI in mental health support

AI is being used more widely in physical health, but it is being adopted more slowly in mental health applications [39]. Mental health professionals are often more dedicated and attentive to their patients' well-being in clinical settings, in contrast to many other non-psychiatric professionals. They prioritize interpersonal skills, such as fostering strong patient relationships and closely monitoring behaviors and emotional responses [40]. Mental health clinical records usually include personal observations and descriptions from patients, along with detailed notes from healthcare providers. However, there remains a significant opportunity for the field of mental health to leverage AI advancements to enhance its practices [41]. AI has the potential to revolutionize the way we diagnose and understand mental illnesses [42]. An individual's unique bio-psycho-social profile is key to understanding their overall mental health [43], but we still have a limited understanding of how these biological, psychological, and social factors interact. Mental illnesses vary greatly in their causes, and finding biomarkers could help define these conditions more clearly and objectively. Using AI techniques can help develop better tools for early screening and create risk models to assess a person's likelihood of developing mental illness [44]. To achieve the long-term goal of personalized mental healthcare, it is essential to utilize computational methods that are most effective for handling big data.

Table 1.7 shows various studies where AI techniques have been used to support mental health, particularly in detecting mental health conditions such as depression, suicide ideation, and medication adherence. It includes different predictors like brain activity, sociological factors, and physical health data.

## 1.6 CHALLENGES

The impact of artificial intelligence on healthcare is profound, offering a variety of advantages, such as more accurate diagnostics, customized treatment strategies, and improved overall patient care. Despite these benefits, incorporating AI into healthcare brings forth a series of challenges that must be carefully considered. These obstacles include concerns over data protection, the need for transparency in algorithms, ethical dilemmas, and the establishment of regulatory policies to ensure the technology's safety and effectiveness. Additionally, there are concerns regarding the dependability of AI systems, the possibility of biased outcomes, and how the roles of healthcare providers might change due to AI integration. In the following, we explore these key challenges in more detail.

### 1.6.1 Data quality and integration

Healthcare data is often fragmented, residing in disparate systems and formats. AI algorithms require large, high-quality datasets for training and validation. However, integrating and harmonizing heterogeneous data sources while ensuring data accuracy, completeness, and relevance poses significant challenges. Poor data quality or biases in training data can adversely affect the performance and reliability of AI models, leading to inaccurate predictions or decisions.

*Table 1.7* Researcher contributions to mental health support

| *References* | *Predictors* | *AI method* | *Performance* |
|---|---|---|---|
| Arun et al. [45] | Mental health, physical weakness, lung capacity, body mass index (BMI), and low-density lipoprotein (LDL) | Supervised machine learning (SML) | XGBoost: accuracy = 98%, sensitivity (SN) = 98%, specificity (SP) = 94% |
| Fernandes et al. [46] | Terms related to suicide in epidemiological studies, records of patients with prior suicide attempts, and recommendations from healthcare professionals. | NLP SML | SVM: suicide ideation SN = 88%, precision = 92%; suicide attempts SN = 98%, precision = 83% |
| Sau and Bhakta [47] | Social and demographic factors along with physical health conditions. | DL | ANN: accuracy = 97%, Area under the curve (AUC) = 0.99 |
| Drysdale et al. [48] | Analysis of neural network interactions between the limbic system and frontostriatal regions using fMRI data. | Unsupervised machine learning (UML) SML | UL: 4-cluster solution SVM: training accuracy = 89%, SN = 84–91%, and SP = 84–93%, test: accuracy = 86% |
| Kalmady et al. [49] | Analyzing regional brain activity and network interactions using fMRI data. | SML | Ensemble model: accuracy = 87% (vs. chance 53%) |
| Patel et al. [50] | MRI data from multiple modalities, including functional connectivity, brain atrophy, tissue integrity, and lesion detection. | SML | ADTree: diagnosis accuracy = 87%, treatment response accuracy = 89% |
| Cai et al. [51] | EEG data collected during a resting state and in response to auditory stimulation. | SML UML | K-nearest neighbourm (KNN): average accuracy = 77% |
| Erguzel et al. [52] | EEG recordings collected over a 12-hour duration. | SML | ANN: AUC = 0.76 (no feature selection), AUC = 0.91 (with feature selection) |

*(Continued)*

*Table 1.7* (Continued) Researcher contributions to mental health support

| *References* | *Predictors* | *AI method* | *Performance* |
|---|---|---|---|
| Bain et al. [53] | Tracking medication compliance through an enhanced version of directly observed therapy. | CompV | Subjects monitored through the AI platform demonstrated a 90% adherence rate, while those tracked by machine learning in mobile direct observation of treatment (mDOT) showed a 72% adherence. |
| Chattopadhyay [54] | Evaluations of specific symptoms by mental health professionals. | SML | Fuzzy neural hybrid model: accuracy = 96% |
| Wahle et al. [55] | Data from smartphones, including accelerometer readings, Wi-Fi signals, and GPS information, used to track movement and activity. | SML | Random forest (RF) accuracy = 62% |
| Aldarwish and Ahmad [56] | Posts from social media platforms such as LiveJournal, Twitter, and Facebook | NLP SML | Naïve bayes (NB): accuracy = 63%, precision = 100%, recall = 58% |
| Deshpande et al. [57] | Unorganized textual data (Tweet) | NLP SML | NB: Precision = 0.836 Accuracy = 83% |
| Mowery et al. [58] | Unorganized textual data (Tweet) | NLP SML | SVM: F1 score = 52 for a tweet with evidence of depression |

### 1.6.2 Interoperability and standardization

The lack of interoperability standards and data-sharing protocols across healthcare systems hinders the seamless exchange and integration of data needed for AI applications. Incompatibilities between electronic health record (EHR) systems, medical devices, and other healthcare technologies impede the scalability and effectiveness of AI-driven solutions. Achieving interoperability requires collaboration among stakeholders to develop and adopt standardized data formats, interfaces, and communication protocols.

### 1.6.3 Regulatory compliance and legal liability

The regulatory landscape for AI in healthcare is complex and evolving. AI-based medical devices and software applications must comply with regulations such as the Food and Drug Administration (FDA) premarket approval requirements and the European Union's Medical Device Regulation (MDR). Ensuring regulatory compliance and navigating legal liabilities associated with AI-driven healthcare solutions, including liability for adverse outcomes or malpractice, present significant challenges for developers, healthcare providers, and regulatory agencies.

### 1.6.4 Algorithmic bias and fairness

AI algorithms have the potential to unintentionally perpetuate or exacerbate biases that exist within the data used for training. This can result in unfair or discriminatory outcomes, particularly in healthcare-related decisions. Biases related to factors such as race, gender, socioeconomic background, or geographical location can impact aspects like diagnosis, treatment, and access to healthcare services. To overcome these challenges, it is crucial to adopt robust data preprocessing techniques, ensure transparency in the design of algorithms, and establish ongoing monitoring and evaluation processes to promote fairness and equity in AI applications.

### 1.6.5 Ethical and privacy concerns

AI raises ethical considerations related to patient autonomy, consent, privacy, and confidentiality. The use of sensitive healthcare data for AI research and applications raises concerns about data privacy, security breaches, and unauthorized access. Protecting patient confidentiality, ensuring informed consent, and mitigating risks of data misuse or unauthorized disclosure are critical ethical imperatives in AI-driven healthcare.

### 1.6.6 Clinical validation and regulatory approval

Validating the clinical efficacy, safety, and effectiveness of AI algorithms in real-world healthcare settings is essential but challenging. Conducting rigorous clinical validation studies, demonstrating clinical utility, and obtaining regulatory approval for AI-driven medical devices or software applications require significant time, resources, and expertise. Additionally, ensuring the generalizability and reliability of AI models across diverse patient populations and healthcare settings is essential for real-world deployment and adoption.

### 1.6.7 Cost and resource constraints

Despite the potential long-term benefits, implementing AI in healthcare entails upfront costs and resource investments. Developing and deploying AI solutions, acquiring necessary infrastructure and technology, and training healthcare professionals incur financial expenses and resource constraints for healthcare organizations. Addressing cost-effectiveness, assessing return on investment, and ensuring equitable access to AI-driven healthcare solutions in resource-limited settings are critical considerations for sustainable implementation.

## 1.7 FUTURE SCOPE

The future scope of artificial intelligence (AI) in healthcare and biomedical science holds significant promise in further transforming the field and improving medical practices globally. AI is expected to continue driving advancements in medical imaging and diagnostics, where it will aid in even earlier detection of diseases, potentially even before symptoms appear. AI will also play a crucial role in enhancing the precision of personalized treatment plans, enabling doctors to tailor interventions to individual patient profiles based on real-time data. In drug discovery, AI's role will expand to include the identification of not only novel drug compounds but also potential drug repurposing opportunities. It is expected that AI models will be able to simulate the interactions between different drugs and patient genetics, helping create highly effective, personalized treatments.

The field of mental health support will benefit from further AI development, with predictive modeling tools advancing the ability to forecast mental health conditions early, offering timely interventions. AI will continue to empower clinicians with personalized recommendations for mental health care, reducing human error and improving patient outcomes. Moreover, AI's contribution to biomedical science will deepen, particularly in areas like genomics, genetic research, and biological data analysis, helping scientists unlock the mysteries of complex biological systems. AI-driven advancements in personalized medicine will lead to treatments based on individual genetic makeup, providing patients with more targeted and effective therapies.

However, for AI to reach its full potential in healthcare, challenges such as data privacy, algorithmic bias, regulatory compliance, and ethical considerations must be addressed. In the future, collaboration between AI experts, healthcare providers, and policymakers will be critical in developing the necessary frameworks for responsible AI use. This will ensure that AI can enhance the quality of care, improve operational efficiency, and ultimately lead to better health outcomes while maintaining ethical standards and patient privacy.

## 1.8 CONCLUSION

As we look ahead to the future of healthcare and biomedical science, the role of AI is becoming increasingly significant. AI is being integrated into various facets of medical research and patient care, reshaping the healthcare field. It has the ability to accelerate drug development, improve diagnostic accuracy, and deliver personalized mental health solutions, offering new approaches to medical challenges. However, it is vital to acknowledge both the benefits and the obstacles that come with this transformation. To ensure AI reaches its full potential, addressing concerns such as data privacy, fairness, and cross-disciplinary collaboration is essential.

In conclusion, artificial intelligence (AI) is playing an increasingly important role in transforming healthcare and biomedical science by offering innovative solutions to some of the most complex challenges. It is making healthcare more accurate, efficient, and accessible, which ultimately benefits patients worldwide. AI is helping doctors and medical professionals by improving medical imaging for early detection of diseases, making drug discovery faster and more precise, and offering personalized care for mental health through predictive models. These advancements make it possible for healthcare providers to offer tailored treatments, improving patient outcomes and reducing side effects. AI is also helping biomedical scientists to better understand the human body, its biological systems, and how genetic information impacts health. This information allows for more precise treatments, such as personalized medicine, which is designed specifically for each patient's needs. Despite these promising developments, the integration of AI into healthcare is not without challenges. Issues such as protecting patient data, minimizing errors in AI algorithms, ensuring fairness, and meeting regulatory standards are significant obstacles that need to be addressed. Additionally, AI systems often rely on large amounts of data, which raises concerns about privacy and bias, making it essential to have strong data governance policies in place.

For AI to continue making a positive impact in healthcare, it is crucial for doctors, researchers, technology developers, and policymakers to work together. They must create clear guidelines and ethical frameworks to ensure that AI is used responsibly and with the best interests of patients in mind. Collaborative efforts will also be necessary to ensure that AI technology is accessible to everyone, regardless of geographical or financial barriers.

The future of artificial intelligence in healthcare and biomedical science holds immense promise. As AI technologies advance, we anticipate quicker diagnoses, enhanced treatment options, and more positive experiences for patients. However, for AI to make a real difference in healthcare, it is crucial to address concerns surrounding ethics, security, and fairness. By ensuring thoughtful planning and responsible deployment, AI can significantly transform healthcare and biomedical fields, ultimately contributing to improved health and extended life expectancy for individuals worldwide.

## REFERENCES


1. Davenport, Thomas H., and Rajeev Ronanki. "Artificial intelligence for the real world." *Harvard Business Review* 96.1 (2018): 108–116.
2. Esteva, Andre, et al. "Dermatologist-level classification of skin cancer with deep neural networks." *Nature* 542.7639 (2017): 115–118.
3. Rajkomar, Alvin, et al. "Scalable and accurate deep learning with electronic health records." *NPJ Digital Medicine* 1.1 (2018): 1–10.
4. Beam, Andrew L., and Isaac S. Kohane. "Translating artificial intelligence into clinical care." *JAMA* 316.22 (2016): 2368–2369.
5. Collins, Francis S., and Harold Varmus. "A new initiative on precision medicine." *New England Journal of Medicine* 372.9 (2015): 793–795.
6. Topol, Eric J. "High-performance medicine: the convergence of human and artificial intelligence." *Nature Medicine* 25.1 (2019): 44–56.
7. Plummer, Susan, and Yasser El Miedany. "Regenerative medicine: challenges and opportunities." *Musculoskeletal Ultrasound-Guided Regenerative Medicine*, 2022, 539–548.
8. Juengst, Eric, et al. "From 'personalized' to 'precision' medicine: the ethical and social implications of rhetorical reform in genomic medicine." *Hastings Center Report* 46.5 (2016): 21–33.
9. Lo, S-CB, et al. "Artificial convolution neural network techniques and applications for lung nodule detection." *IEEE Transactions on Medical Imaging* 14.4 (1995): 711–718.
10. Ronneberger, Olaf, Philipp Fischer, and Thomas Brox. "U-net: convolutional networks for biomedical image segmentation." Medical Image Computing and Computer-Assisted Intervention–MICCAI 2015: 18th International Conference, Munich, Germany, October 5–9, 2015, proceedings, part III 18. Springer International Publishing, 2015.
11. Dou, Qi, et al. "Automatic detection of cerebral microbleeds from MR images via 3D convolutional neural networks." *IEEE Transactions on Medical Imaging* 35.5 (2016): 1182–1195.
12. Yu, Lequan, et al. "Automated melanoma recognition in dermoscopy images via very deep residual networks." *IEEE Transactions on Medical Imaging* 36.4 (2016): 994–1004.
13. Lao, Jiangwei, et al. "A deep learning-based radiomics model for prediction of survival in glioblastoma multiforme." *Scientific Reports* 7.1 (2017): 10353.
14. Kamnitsas, Konstantinos, et al. "Efficient multi-scale 3D CNN with fully connected CRF for accurate brain lesion segmentation." *Medical Image Analysis* 36 (2017): 61–78.
15. Zhu, Zhe, et al. "Deep learning for identifying radiogenomic associations in breast cancer." *Computers in Biology and Medicine* 109 (2019): 85–90.
16. Chartsias, Agisilaos, et al. "Factorised spatial representation learning: application in semi-supervised myocardial segmentation." Medical Image Computing and Computer Assisted Intervention–MICCAI 2018: 21st International Conference, Granada, Spain, September 16–20, 2018, Proceedings, Part II 11. Springer International Publishing, 2018.
17. McKinney, Scott Mayer, et al. "International evaluation of an AI system for breast cancer screening." *Nature* 577.7788 (2020): 89–94.

18. Hekler, Achim, et al. "Pathologist-level classification of histopathological melanoma images with deep neural networks." *European Journal of Cancer* 115 (2019): 79–83.
19. Vamathevan, Jessica, et al. "Applications of machine learning in drug discovery and development." *Nature Reviews Drug Discovery* 18.6 (2019): 463–477.
20. Lavecchia, Antonio. "Machine-learning approaches in drug discovery: methods and applications." *Drug Discovery Today* 20.3 (2015): 318–331.
21. Schmidhuber, Jürgen. "Deep learning in neural networks: an overview." *Neural Networks* 61 (2015): 85–117.
22. Xue, Ling, and Jurgen Bajorath. "Molecular descriptors in chemoinformatics, computational combinatorial chemistry, and virtual screening." *Combinatorial Chemistry & High Throughput Screening* 3.5 (2000): 363–372.
23. Schneider, Gisbert. "Mind and machine in drug design." *Nature Machine Intelligence* 1.3 (2019): 128–130.
24. Wu, Zhenqin, et al. "Molecule net: a benchmark for molecular machine learning." *Chemical Science* 9.2 (2018): 513–530.
25. Feinberg, Evan N., et al. "Potential net for molecular property prediction." *ACS Central Science* 4.11 (2018): 1520–1530.
26. Jumper, John, et al. "Highly accurate protein structure prediction with Alpha fold." *Nature* 596.7873 (2021): 583–589.
27. Ramsundar, Bharath. *Molecular machine learning with DeepChem*. Diss. Stanford University, 2018.
28. Alipanahi, Babak, et al. "Predicting the sequence specificities of DNA-and RNA-binding proteins by deep learning." *Nature Biotechnology* 33.8 (2015): 831–838.
29. Ding, Xinqiang, and Bin Zhang. "DeepBAR: a fast and exact method for binding free energy computation." *The Journal of Physical Chemistry Letters* 12.10 (2021): 2509–2515.
30. Liu, Zhihong, et al. "DeepScreening: a deep learning-based screening web server for accelerating drug discovery." *Database* 2019 (2019): baz104.
31. Rifaioglu, Ahmet Sureyya, et al. "DEEPScreen: high performance drug–target interaction prediction with convolutional neural networks using 2-D structural compound representations." *Chemical Science* 11.9 (2020): 2531–2557.
32. Lee, Ingoo, Jongsoo Keum, and Hojung Nam. "DeepConv-DTI: prediction of drug-target interactions via deep learning with convolution on protein sequences." *PLoS Computational Biology* 15.6 (2019): e1007129.
33. Huang, Kexin, et al. "DeepPurpose: a deep learning library for drug–target interaction prediction." *Bioinformatics* 36.22–23 (2020): 5545–5547.
34. Mayr, Andreas, et al. "DeepTox: toxicity prediction using deep learning." *Frontiers in Environmental Science* 3 (2016): 80.
35. Wallach, Izhar, Michael Dzamba, and Abraham Heifets. "AtomNet: a deep convolutional neural network for bioactivity prediction in structure-based drug discovery." *arXiv preprint arXiv:1510.02855* (2015).
36. Tang, Yi-Ching, and Assaf Gottlieb. "Explainable drug sensitivity prediction through cancer pathway enrichment." *Scientific Reports* 11.1 (2021): 3128.
37. Gómez-Bombarelli, Rafael, et al. "Automatic chemical design using a data-driven continuous representation of molecules." *ACS Central Science* 4.2 (2018): 268–276.

38. Zhu, Zhaocheng, et al. "Torchdrug: a powerful and flexible machine learning platform for drug discovery." *arXiv preprint arXiv:2202.08320* (2022).
39. Jiang, Fei, et al. "Artificial intelligence in healthcare: past, present and future." *Stroke and Vascular Neurology* 2.4 (2017):,230–243.
40. Gabbard, Glen O., and Holly Crisp-Han. "The early career psychiatrist and the psychotherapeutic identity." *Academic Psychiatry* 41 (2017): 30–34.
41. Janssen, Ronald J., Janaina Mourão-Miranda, and Hugo G. Schnack. "Making individual prognoses in psychiatry using neuroimaging and machine learning." *Biological Psychiatry: Cognitive Neuroscience and Neuroimaging* 3.9 (2018): 798–808.
42. Bzdok, Danilo, and Andreas Meyer-Lindenberg. "Machine learning for precision psychiatry: opportunities and challenges." *Biological Psychiatry: Cognitive Neuroscience and Neuroimaging* 3.3 (2018): 223–230.
43. Jeste, Dilip V., et al. "Study of independent living residents of a continuing care senior housing community: sociodemographic and clinical associations of cognitive, physical, and mental health." *The American Journal of Geriatric Psychiatry* 27.9 (2019): 895–907.
44. Shatte, Adrian BR, Delyse M. Hutchinson, and Samantha J. Teague. "Machine learning in mental health: a scoping review of methods and applications." *Psychological Medicine* 49.9 (2019): 1426–1448.
45. Arun, Vanishri, et al. "A boosted machine learning approach for detection of depression." 2018 IEEE Symposium Series on Computational Intelligence (SSCI). IEEE, 2018.
46. Fernandes, Andrea C., et al. "Identifying suicide ideation and suicidal attempts in a psychiatric clinical research database using natural language processing." *Scientific Reports* 8.1 (2018): 7426.
47. Sau, Arkaprabha, and Ishita Bhakta. "Artificial neural network (ANN) model to predict depression among geriatric population at a slum in Kolkata, India." *Journal of Clinical and Diagnostic Research: JCDR* 11.5 (2017): VC01.
48. Drysdale, Andrew T., et al. "Resting-state connectivity biomarkers define neurophysiological subtypes of depression." *Nature Medicine* 23.1 (2017): 28–38.
49. Kalmady, Sunil Vasu, et al. "Towards artificial intelligence in mental health by improving schizophrenia prediction with multiple brain parcellation ensemble-learning." *NPJ Schizophrenia* 5.1 (2019): 2.
50. Patel, Meenal J., et al. "Machine learning approaches for integrating clinical and imaging features in late-life depression classification and response prediction." *International Journal of Geriatric Psychiatry* 30.10 (2015): 1056–1067.
51. Cai, Hanshu, et al. "A pervasive approach to EEG-based depression detection." *Complexity* 2018.1 (2018): 5238028.
52. Erguzel, Turker Tekin, Gokben Hizli Sayar, and Nevzat Tarhan. "Artificial intelligence approach to classify unipolar and bipolar depressive disorders." *Neural Computing and Applications* 27.6 (2016): 1607–1616.
53. Bain, Earle E., et al. "Use of a novel artificial intelligence platform on mobile devices to assess dosing compliance in a phase 2 clinical trial in subjects with schizophrenia." JMIR mHealth and uHealth 5.2 (2017): e7030.
54. Chattopadhyay, Subhagata. "A neuro-fuzzy approach for the diagnosis of depression." *Applied Computing and Informatics* 13.1 (2017): 10–18.

55. Wahle, Fabian, et al. "Mobile sensing and support for people with depression: a pilot trial in the wild." *JMIR mHealth and uHealth* 4.3 (2016): e5960.
56. Aldarwish, Maryam Mohammed, and Hafiz Farooq Ahmad. "Predicting depression levels using social media posts." 2017 IEEE 13th International Symposium on Autonomous Decentralized System (ISADS). IEEE, 2017.
57. Deshpande, Mandar, and Vignesh Rao. "Depression detection using emotion artificial intelligence." 2017 international Conference on Intelligent Sustainable Systems (ICISS). IEEE, 2017.
58. Mowery, Danielle L., et al. "Towards automatically classifying depressive symptoms from Twitter data for population health." Proceedings of the Workshop on Computational Modeling of People's Opinions, Personality, and Emotions in Social Media (PEOPLES), 2016.

Chapter 2

# Applications of artificial intelligence in healthcare

*Rashmi Rameshwari, Naina Soni, Devendra Kumar Verma, and Santosh Kumar*

## 2.1 INTRODUCTION

Artificial intelligence (AI) and data science have seen significant technological advancements over the last decade. Despite a decades-long history of AI research, the current spike in AI excitement differs significantly from previous epochs. This disparity is due to an optimum combination of increased computer processing capabilities, large data aggregation repositories, and a growing pool of AI knowledge. These combined elements have accelerated the progress of AI techniques, particularly in the healthcare industry. Due to this convergence, a significant change in the complexity of AI technologies is anticipated, significantly changing their adoption and impact on social systems.[1] AI has advanced dramatically since Christopher Strachey created the inaugural AI program in 1951. Initially confined to academic research, the inception of modern AI can be traced back to John McCarthy's seminal 1956 Dartmouth Conference, which formally coined the term "artificial intelligence" and catalyzed a paradigm shift in computational thought. Subsequent decades witnessed a progressive evolution—from symbolic reasoning in the 1960s to the advent of machine learning and neural architectures in the 1980s and 1990s—culminating in the landmark 1997 triumph of IBM's Deep Blue over chess grandmaster Garry Kasparov, a pivotal moment in AI's ascendancy. In the 2000s, AI continued to advance with a focus on natural language processing (NLP) and computer vision (Figure 2.1). This advancement resulted in the development of virtual assistants such as Apple's Siri and Amazon's Alexa, which can interpret and interact with human speech.[2,3] AI research initially focused on rule-based expert systems, but its progress was significantly impeded by the limitations in computational power and the scarcity of accessible data. The emergence of deep learning (DL) has profoundly transformed our knowledge of AI tools and is a significant contributor to the current surge of interest in AI applications. Deep learning allows for detecting complex patterns and correlations previously impossible with traditional machine learning methods. This achievement has revolutionized the AI environment, enabling the creation of more advanced and competent solutions in


DOI: 10.1201/9781003741770-2

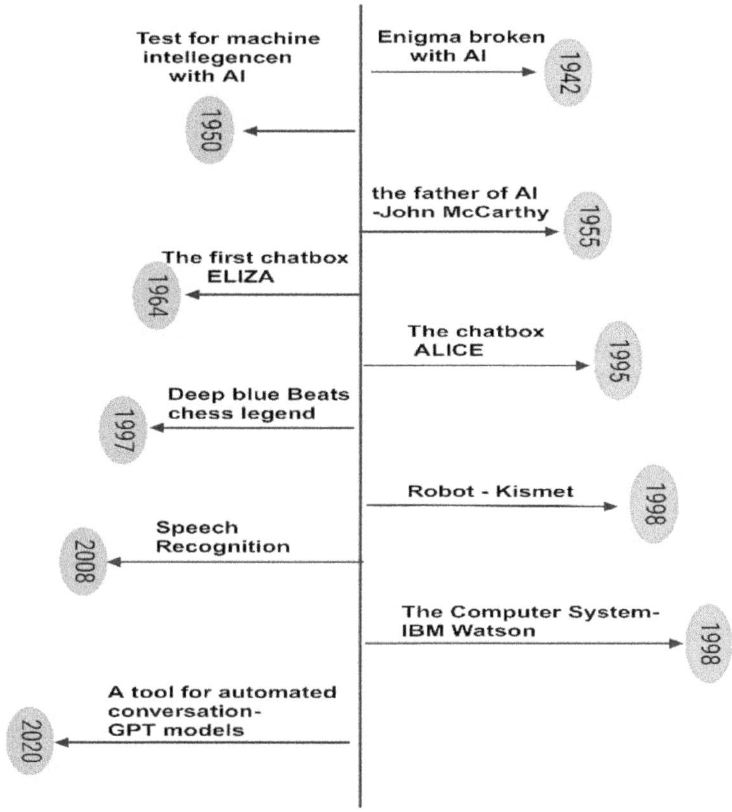


*Figure 2.1* The chart shows the progression of AI over the years

various disciplines. Leading businesses in this space include IBM Watson and Google DeepMind. IBM Watson and Google's DeepMind are widely used in various healthcare applications, demonstrating the vast potential of AI in medicine. IBM Watson is working on multiple topics, including diabetes treatment, improved cancer care and modeling, and drug development. Despite its unique capabilities, Watson has failed to provide meaningful clinical advantages to patients.

DeepMind, on the other hand, is being studied for various healthcare applications, including serving as a mobile medical assistant, improving diagnoses through medical imaging, and forecasting patient deterioration. These projects show the continuous research of AI technology and its use to improve patient care and medical results.[4] AI tools are set to enhance, not replace, the work of healthcare professionals. They facilitate administrative processes, streamline clinical documentation, and improve patient engagement while offering specialized expertise in imaging analysis, automation of medical devices, and continuous patient monitoring. This enables healthcare professionals to redirect their efforts toward nuanced clinical judgment and direct patient engagement. Divergent viewpoints persist concerning the most efficacious and impactful utilizations of AI within the medical sphere. According to a Forbes report (2018), critical areas of AI integration include optimizing administrative workflows, advancing imaging analysis, enhancing robotic surgery, deploying virtual assistants, and bolstering clinical decision-making processes.[5] Then, a 2019 report by McKinsey identifies critical areas where AI can significantly impact healthcare, including the emergence of intelligent, interconnected devices, the advancement of precision therapeutics, the augmentation of robotic surgery, and the innovation of electroceuticals.[6] The healthcare sector is progressively recognizing AI-infused technologies' profound transformative capacity in redefining the contours of future medical methodologies. AI is set to revolutionize various facets of healthcare operations and service delivery, with projected cost savings in the US healthcare system anticipated to reach USD 150 billion annually by 2026. These savings are primarily attributed to a shift toward proactive health management, which aims to reduce hospital admissions, physician consultations, and treatment interventions. AI technologies facilitate continuous monitoring, personalized therapeutic approaches, and efficient follow-up care, enabling earlier diagnoses and improved health outcomes. The AI-driven healthcare sector is anticipated to undergo rapid proliferation, with estimations foreseeing its valuation reaching USD 6.6 billion by 2021, underpinned by an exceptional compound annual growth trajectory of 40%. The ensuing sections will delve into pivotal AI applications within healthcare, encompassing its direct clinical implementations and its integrative role across domains such as diagnostic innovation, pharmacological development, and ambient-assisted living (AAL) within the broader healthcare continuum.

## 2.2 AI'S ROLE IN DIAGNOSTIC ASSISTANCE

Rapid identification of infectious diseases and prompt containment measures rely on continuous data analysis. The efficiency and efficacy of these efforts significantly impact global social welfare and economic stability.[6] Despite significant progress in medical science, the accurate diagnosis of diseases persists as a formidable global impediment, further compounded by the convoluted etiology of ailments and the polymorphism of clinical manifestations. This intrinsic complexity hinders the evolution of robust early diagnostic frameworks. Nonetheless, the integration of artificial intelligence (AI), particularly through the deployment of machine learning (ML) algorithms, holds the potential to radically recalibrate the diagnostic paradigm, heralding a transformative epoch in medical practice.[7] ML algorithms improve diagnostic accuracy by utilizing data, which is influenced by the quantity and quality of input data, addressing some of the inherent complexities and challenges associated with diagnosis. This section delves into critical machine learning-based disease diagnoses (MLBD).[8] In light of the widespread impact of COVID-19, research since 2020 has focused on detecting the disease using ML, which is currently a significant area of investigation. This section also provides a comprehensive discussion of heart disease, diabetes, and COVID-19.

### 2.2.1 Heart diseases

Machine learning (ML) methodologies are frequently utilized by researchers and clinicians in cardiac disease diagnostics. In a notable study, Ansari et al.[9] proposed a sophisticated algorithmic diagnostic architecture tailored for the autonomous detection of coronary heart disease, marking a pivotal advancement in computational cardiology, employing a neurofuzzy integrated system, reporting an accuracy of approximately 89%. Nevertheless, this study lacks sufficient detail in delineating the system's efficacy across various scenarios, including multiclass classification challenges, extensive datasets, and imbalanced class distributions. Furthermore, it neglects to substantiate the credibility of the model's accuracy, an increasingly emphasized criterion in medical domains to facilitate comprehension and trust among non-expert users.[9,10] Researchers employed deep convolutional neural networks to identify abnormal cardiac sounds. By strategically calibrating the loss function to enhance sensitivity and specificity across the training dataset concurrently, the model exhibited robust discriminative capability. Its efficacy was substantiated in the 2016 PhysioNet Computing Challenge, where it secured an impressive second-place standing, attaining a specificity of 0.95 and a sensitivity of 0.73.[11] In another realm, recent attention has focused on deep learning (DL) algorithms for cardiac disease detection. For example, researchers devised a deep learning (DL) methodology for fetal health diagnosis using cardiotocographic data. This approach effectively differentiates and classifies morphologic patterns linked to pregnancy complications. The initial computational metrics revealed a classification accuracy of 88.02%, a precision rate of 85.01%, and an F1-score converging at 0.85, collectively underscoring the model's robust predictive efficacy and balanced performance across evaluative dimensions. The study incorporated various dropout techniques to mitigate overfitting, recognizing that the extended training duration was an acceptable compromise for achieving enhanced accuracy.[11] Despite widespread adoption in heart disease diagnosis, current ML applications still need to adequately address challenges related to unbalanced data in multiclass classification and explain model decisions sufficiently during final predictions.[12]

### 2.2.2 Diabetes

Diabetes poses a formidable challenge in the global healthcare landscape, ranked by the World Health Organization (WHO) as the seventh most common cause of premature mortality in 2016.[13] Annually, it claims the lives of 1.6 million individuals worldwide. From 1980 to 2014, the incidence of diabetes escalated dramatically, increasing from 108 million to 422 million cases. The escalating incidence is compounded by a rising epidemic of obesity, affecting approximately one-third of adults globally. Diabetes is intricately associated with severe health ramifications such as heart attacks, kidney failure, stroke, and blindness.[14] A substantial body of empirical research has substantiated the diagnostic proficiency of machine learning (ML) paradigms in the identification of diabetes mellitus. Notably, investigators have conducted comparative assessments of diverse classification algorithms—including J48 decision trees (DTs), k-nearest neighbors (KNNs), random forests (RFs), and support vector machines (SVMs)—applied to the UCI Diabetes dataset. Among these, the KNN algorithm configured with K = 1K = 1K = 1, alongside the RF classifier, demonstrated near-optimal diagnostic precision, approaching the upper bounds of classification accuracy.[15–16] However, a limitation is using a simplified dataset with only eight binary parameters, which may overstate accuracy. The studies also warrant a more comprehensive analysis of how algorithmic predictions are translated for non-specialist audiences. Additionally, another investigation implemented clinical decision support systems (CDSSs) for diabetes diagnosis, employing support vector machines (SVMs), random forests (RFs), and deep convolutional neural networks (CNNs). Among these methodologies, RF exhibited the most robust performance, attaining a classification accuracy of 83.67%. The KNN algorithm outperformed its counterparts, with deep learning (DL) and support vector machines (SVMs) registering comparatively lower accuracies of 76.81% and 65.38%, respectively. Subsequently, scholars extended their analytical scope by deploying an array of machine learning methodologies—such as artificial neural networks (ANNs), naïve Bayes (NB), decision trees (DTs), and deep learning (DL)—to interrogate the PIMA Indian Diabetes dataset, further elucidating the predictive capabilities of these computational frameworks in metabolic disorder diagnostics. DL emerged as the most accurate method, achieving approximately 98.07% accuracy in predicting diabetes development. While the PIMA dataset is well-studied and facilitates the application of conventional and advanced ML algorithms, the study overlooks interpretability issues and the model's performance on unbalanced or incomplete datasets—a critical consideration in healthcare where data labeling and preprocessing can vary significantly.[17] Researchers addressed overfitting in the PIMA Indian dataset using deep learning, achieving 88.41% accuracy with dropout techniques.[18] They also presented a clinical decision support system (CDSS) framework applied to the King Abdullah International Research

Center for Diabetes dataset, which achieved accuracy levels up to 97% utilizing deep neural networks based on long short-term memory (LSTM) and gated recurrent unit architectures.[19] The findings underscore artificial intelligence's substantial prognostic and diagnostic potential in elucidating diabetic complications, with far-reaching implications for enhancing clinical outcomes and augmenting the economic efficiency of diabetes management paradigms.

### 2.2.3 COVID-19

Initially detected in China in December 2019, COVID-19 was officially declared a Public Health Emergency of International Concern in January 2020, subsequently escalating to the status of a global pandemic, as proclaimed by the WHO on March 11, 2020.[20] Vaccines for COVID-19 have been promptly produced and are currently being administered globally to mitigate the impact of the disease.[21] However, issues such as missability, altered antigenicity, and potential reductions in immunity may affect vaccination effectiveness. Therapeutic interventions for COVID-19 are being developed and authorized, including remdesivir, dexamethasone, and baricitinib, which are being utilized in clinical practice.[22,23] Significantly, research on COVID-19 is being conducted globally, with AI playing a crucial role in accelerating advancements in vaccine development, creating novel diagnostic techniques, and discovering new therapeutic agents.[24] By analyzing vast datasets, AI enables identifying key features critical to these developments. Here, the discussion is focused on the current state of AI applications in developing COVID-19 vaccines, innovative diagnostic methods, and therapeutic interventions. It also discusses AI's pivotal role in addressing the challenges posed by the pandemic. Amid the COVID-19 pandemic, AI has emerged as a pivotal force in refining chest X-ray image analysis for diagnosis and therapeutic decision-making. Researchers have meticulously adapted pre-trained convolutional models such as ResNet and DenseNet121 for the nuanced detection of COVID-19[7] while addressing the challenges of limited data through the implementation of a patch-based CNN integrated with gradient-weighted class activation mapping (Grad-CAM) to enhance interpretability.[25] Furthermore, weakly supervised learning architectures have been leveraged to intricately assess the severity of pulmonary compromise, with the DenseNet121 model notably demonstrating prognostic efficacy in anticipating the early requirement for mechanical ventilation.[26] These sophisticated AI methodologies provide profound insights into the subtle dynamics of disease progression and patient management.[27] Rapid advancements in COVID-19 vaccine and drug discovery are driven by AI and deep learning (DL) technologies. DL models have been instrumental in identifying therapeutic antibodies through antigen specificity prediction, with the MARIA framework aiding epitope prediction using human leukocyte antigen-DR (HLA-DR) ligand data.[27] Deep neural networks (DNNs) are utilized for antibody-epitope classification, and the REDIAL-2020 ML platform assesses compound activities related to severe acute respiratory syndrome coronavirus 2 (SARS-CoV-2).[28] ML-based pipelines are also being developed to uncover effective COVID-19 therapies from existing drugs.

In silico drug discovery, tensor decomposition has successfully identified compounds such as ivermectin. Fragment-based drug discovery has identified lead compounds, while drug repurposing has utilized protein–protein interaction networks and matrix completion techniques.[29] AI-driven platforms are increasingly used for drug screening and mortality prediction across various populations.[30] The COVID-19 Moonshot endeavor represents a paradigmatic fusion of academic insight and industrial capability, mobilized to expedite the rational design of inhibitors against the SARS-CoV-2 main protease (Mpro). This initiative harnesses a multifaceted strategy, interweaving decentralized crowdsourced ideation, ultra-high-throughput crystallographic analyses, algorithmically intensive computational chemistry, and machine learning algorithms to accelerate the antiviral discovery pipeline.[31] Historical epidemics have demonstrated that the complete eradication of pathogenic viruses is improbable due to ongoing mutations and the emergence of drug resistance. Consequently, it is imperative to remain attuned to the latest developments in viral infection management. The deployment of AI in combating COVID-19 confers significant advantages, notably expediting the development of vaccines and therapeutics while enhancing the precision and efficiency of diagnostic methodologies. Additionally, the integration of explainable AI can enhance clinical decision-making within hospitals, promoting broader adoption and improving healthcare outcomes.[32]

## 2.3 AI'S ROLE IN UNRAVELING DRUG DEVELOPMENT COMPLEXITIES

In the convoluted domain of treating multifactorial diseases, the synthesis of combination therapies has become paramount. Monotherapeutic approaches often prove inadequate, failing to engage the diverse and critical therapeutic targets necessary for holistic intervention. Consider cancer therapy, where patients may harbor multiple molecular aberrations in their genomic profiles. Here lies the need for combining drugs synergistically to achieve optimal outcomes.[33] Historically, the concept of drug synergy dates back to Loewe's classical work in 1928, which continues to inform calculations for optimal drug combinations. However, recent years have witnessed an explosion of information. For drugs, hundreds of 2D and 3D molecular descriptors are now available. Simultaneously, patient data have expanded to include genetic, proteomic, and metabolomic profiles alongside traditional clinical information. However, the complexity continues to increase. Disease progression alters genetic profiles, making it challenging for individual physicians to comprehend and optimize drug combinations for each patient. Biomedical informatics and artificial intelligence (AI) offer solutions beyond human capacity, enabling personalized drug regimens tailored to each patient's needs. As we embrace AI, the future of combination therapies becomes increasingly precise and patient-centered.[34]

## 2.4 ADVANCING DRUG DISCOVERY: THE SYNERGY OF ARTIFICIAL INTELLIGENCE AND CONVENTIONAL CHEMISTS

In the evolving realm of pharmaceutical research, artificial intelligence (AI) has emerged as an innovative approach to addressing the enduring challenges of classical chemistry and chemical space, which frequently obstruct the progress of drug discovery and development. Technological progress and high-performance computing have profoundly amplified the impact of AI—ranging from ML to DL—in revolutionizing computer-aided drug design.[35] Although AI is not a novel concept within drug research, chemists persist in their quest for precise predictions of chemical activity–structure relationships.

Historically, figures such as Hammett and Hansch laid foundational work in this field. Hammett linked reaction kinetics to equilibrium constants, while Hansch pioneered computational approaches to forecast drug compounds' physicochemical traits and bioactivity.[35] Hansch's pioneering achievements catalyzed subsequent investigations, which concentrated on two pivotal areas.

### 2.4.1 Detailed identification and prediction

Researchers strive to accurately delineate chemical structures and elucidate properties such as pharmacophores and three-dimensional conformations. This endeavor entails the application of advanced mathematical formulations that establish correlations between chemical representations and biological activity.

- **ML algorithms and classical chemistry:** In today's scientific milieu, the principal aim is to enhance the accuracy and dependability of drug discovery methodologies. Machine learning (ML) algorithms, firmly anchored in classical chemical principles, are integral to this mission. They address fundamental inquiries in medicinal chemistry, including "Which compound is most advantageous?" and, following this, "What is the optimal synthesis strategy?[35, 36]

Different methods and instruments have been developed for computerized drug exploration in the last twenty years. Some significant methods include the following:

- **Quantitative structure–activity relationship (QSAR) methods:** These models correlate molecular structures with biological activity, aiding in compound prediction.[34]
- **Free-energy minimization techniques:** Optimize molecular conformations and interactions, which are crucial for drug binding.

Recent research highlights the transformative impact of AI in drug discovery:

**Prediction of compound-cell activity:** Sophisticated AI models, such as DTs, RFs, CNNs, SVMs, LSTMs, and gradient boosting, are leveraged to predict compound-cell interactions, often using simplified molecular input line entry system (SMILES) strings akin to NLP inputs, enabling accurate classification of cellular activity across diverse compounds.

**Prediction of PAMPA effective permeability:** A dual QSAR approach fuses classical QSAR modeling with machine learning-driven techniques for enhanced predictive accuracy. Within this paradigm, hierarchical support vector machines (SVMs) have been shown to surpass partial least squares in both the training and testing phases.

**Screening hepatotoxic ingredients:** Computational techniques identify hepatotoxic compounds in traditional Chinese medicines.[37]

**Novel coronavirus research:** Computational methods screen bioactive compounds targeting SARS with precision. Existing Chinese traditional medicines show promise.[38]

In this symbiotic endeavor, chemical scientists collaborate with computational experts to develop modern ML algorithms. The fusion of classical chemistry and AI holds immense potential for future drug discovery and development. As they unravel the complexities of biological systems, this interdisciplinary approach shapes the pharmaceutical landscape. Moving further with the advancement of AI in healthcare, precision medicine is another emerging field that provides the utmost promising patient care.

## 2.5 PRECISION MEDICINE: A CUSTOMIZED, FLEXIBLE FRAMEWORK

Precision medicine, often known as personalized medicine, represents a paradigm change in healthcare. Individual heterogeneity in environment, genes, and lifestyle is considered to customize disease treatment and preventive measures for each person. Despite the traditional one-size-fits-all approach, precision medicine considers each person unique. It seeks to anticipate which therapies will be most effective for specific groups based on their genetic composition, environment, and lifestyle choices. In essence, personalized medicine uses molecular biology findings, such as genome sequencing, to transform how we view health and well-being. Rather than relying merely on generalizations, it strives to deliver tailored, customized care that enhances efficacy while minimizing danger.[39]

Precision medicine empowers healthcare practitioners to access and disseminate insights that either reinforce or recalibrate medical decisions, shifting from evidence-based protocols designed for the average patient to strategies tailored to an individual's distinctive characteristics. This approach facilitates the provision of highly personalized care, aligning treatment with the specific nuances of each patient. The discovery of precision medicine uncovers avenues of intervention that might otherwise remain unexplored.

Recent developments in precision medicine have practical advantages, such as early disease identification and the development of individualized therapies, which are becoming increasingly frequent in healthcare.[40,41] A diverse array of data collection methodologies and analytical instruments underpins the capacity of precision medicine to customize patient care. The synergistic integration of high-throughput genotyping and the global proliferation of electronic health records (EHRs) empowers researchers to discern novel phenotypes from clinical and biomarker datasets. When these phenotypes are cross-referenced with EHR data, they can substantiate the necessity for adjunctive pharmacological interventions or refine the diagnostic accuracy of disease subtypes.

Home monitoring and wearable gadgets are transforming diseasedisease detection by allowing non-invasive applications to track health issues such as diabetes, epilepsy, pain management, Parkinson's, cardiovascular disease, sleep disorders, and obesity.[42] Digital biomarkers allow for remote disease monitoring, aiding decentralized clinical studies. In cancer care, wearable technologies use continuous tumor cell analysis to detect minimal residual disease and track its progression.[43–45]

AI and precision medicine research attempt to improve health-related activities by providing individualized diagnostic information, hence increasing early disease identification and prevention. This collaboration might lower the burden of disease and healthcare expenses for the general public.

## 2.6 AI IN HEALTH DIAGNOSIS: OPPORTUNITIES AND ISSUES FOR PRACTICAL PURPOSES

In this chapter, some of the important applications of AI, along with their associated issues, have been discussed. These are as follows:

(a) **AI applications in medical imaging:** Detection of diabetic retinopathy using retinal fundus images; dermatological classification of skin cancer; and data issues.
(b) **Translating computational advances into clinical practice:** Coronary artery disease—issues driving interest; development of new approaches—non-invasive diagnostics; and development and validation for clinical applications.
(c) Evolution of standards for AI in medical applications.

## 2.6 AI APPLICATION FOR MEDICAL IMAGING

In patients with diabetes, it is very important to detect early symptoms of eye diseases. Early detection of symptoms can help prevent the risk of eye vision loss and blindness. These early symptoms can be detected by using non-invasive imaging of the retina through the pupil. Such a type of screening also provides the opportunity for early detection of symptoms of eye disease as well as cardiovascular disease. In routine imaging, fundus cameras are used to capture different images at different orientations, but the assessment of these images needs well-skilled readers and remote specialists. By using digital photography, digital recording of retinal image can be achieved using a picture achieving and communication system. Recently, a deep learning algorithm has been used for retinal image analysis. It was found that this algorithm provides improved quality of outcomes with greater accessibility. It was also concluded that it provides rapid and cost-effective analysis compared to manual assessment, enhancing diagnostic capabilities.

### 2.6.1 Classification of skin cancer

Seventy-five percent of deaths from skin cancer are due to melanoma, even though melanoma accounts for only 3–5% for total skin cancer cases, with 1.5 million cases diagnosed per year in the US. Early detection of melanoma is critical to addressing these health issues. Even with screening exams, limitations exist. The sensitivity and specificity of melanoma detection have been found to be 49% and 97%, respectively, by dermatologists, while for physicians, these values reduce to 40% and 86%, respectively.[46]

In recent studies, convolutional neural network (CNN) algorithms have been used for the detection of melanoma using thousands of dermatologist-labeled images based on biopsy results.[47]

It was concluded that the algorithm performs similarly to or slightly better than individual dermatologists. However, further work is still required to validate the algorithm with different types of samples.

On this basis, two findings emerged: (a) AI algorithms can be applied to medical image analysis based on the capacity of the available medical data, and (b) AI algorithms were found to perform at the standard of the training data and not beyond it.

Overall, one major issue lies with the data. It is a big task to obtain high-quality labeled images to apply AI algorithms. Sometimes, it has been found that the data is obtained in small quantities, and the time required for this data is also insufficient to achieve highly accurate results. Additionally, the data labeled by clinicians is of variable standards and may not be suitable for producing standard results.

### 2.6.2 Other major applications[48–64]

1. Medical diagnosis
2. Robot-assisted surgery
3. Clinical trial
4. Training
5. Fraud detection
6. Drug discovery
7. Stock management
8. Cardial tissue chips
9. Artificial neurons
10. Plastic surgery
11. Organ transplantation
12. Spinal cord injury

The latest application of AI has been used during COVID-19 detection. This application was used to detect a COVID-19 patient by voice-based diagnosis. The Patil Institute of Biotechnology and Bioinformatics, Mumbai, India, has invented a voice-based diagnosis using a mobile phone. The project was a collaborative effort by a team of three students and one professor. This Indian-made voice-based diagnosis gadget for COVID-19 detection has already been used in Italy. The University of Rome reported a 98 percent precision while using this technology to detect COVID-19 patients. The principle behind this instrument is that COVID-19 affects lung function, and as the function changes, the voice coming through the lungs also changes. The patient has to speak into the speaker of the phone. Then the phone analyzes its sound and amplifies it. The voice of a normal human was also recorded for comparison. Hence, it easily detects the patients.[65]

## 2.7 COMPUTATIONAL ADVANCES INTO CLINICAL PRACTICE

Basically, computational analysis is a special type of tool used in different medical practices. However, due to the lack of sufficient validation and experience required for medical practices, these tools have not been extensively used. In this section, we aim to discuss how AI tools can improve clinical practices, making them more effective and cost-efficient.

In many cases, patients who have chest pain undergo invasive testing and receive a negative diagnosis. This not only creates a negative impact on the patient but also represents an expensive method of diagnosis, highlighting the need for an alternate approach.

There are two possibilities to have coronary artery disease: one is that the artery is narrow (stenosis), and the second is that the blood flow is slow in the blood vessels (ischemia). Invasive coronary angiography is performed for the diagnosis of stenosis by injecting a dye into the arteries of the heart, which is visualized using X-ray imaging.

But it is important to notice that more than 60% patients who do not have coronary artery disease (CAD) and 50% of the patients who do not have significantly impaired blood flow have been sent for invasive coronary angiography and revascularization.[66–68]

Therefore, new approaches are required, such as coronary computed tomographic angiography (CCTA), which is a non-invasive diagnostic technique. Recently, computational fluid dynamics with CCTA has been utilized to assess fluid flow reserve computationally. These results reduce the need for the invasive approach.

## 2.8 STANDARDS FOR AI IN MEDICAL APPLICATIONS

AI standards are controlled by FDA and clinical models. Non-clinical smart devices have been used based on public confidence and may or may not fall under regulation. Fractional flow reverse calculated from computed tomography (FFRCT) computational tools have been controlled by the FDA, and for their use, clinical studies are required.[68]

The FDA not only controls clinical models but also pays attention to the global development of software in medical devices (SiMD) and software as a medical device (SaMD). The FDA also chairs both international forums for SiMD and SaMD. The FDA creates and proposes new policies in this forum for SiMD and SaMD.[69–73]

### 2.8.1 Devices and apps for the data collection

The American Medical Association (AMA) recently adopted a set of principles to promote safe and effective mHealth applications. According to an AMA review, physicians and clinical trainers are eager to use these AI and digital tools for efficiency, patient safety, improved diagnostic ability, and improved physician–patient relationships. The three to four most important considerations for their use include data privacy assurance, the ability to link with electronic health records, and billing/reimbursements. The following is a list of some tools used for modern health monitoring.

#### 2.8.1.1 Personal Electrocardiogram (EKG)

This is an FDA-cleared personal EKG recording device. It has a finger pad and a smartphone app that is used to record a 30-second EKG recording. There is no use of wire and gels for operating this device.

#### 2.8.1.2 Parkinson's tremors

To investigate Parkinson's disease symptoms, a new app called CloudUPDRS, which is a smartphone app, has been proposed. This tool enables Parkinson's patients to perform in-home testing, providing valuable and quantitative feedback on how their personal lifestyle factors and medications may affect their symptoms.

#### 2.8.1.3 Asthma tracking and control app

This app is used to monitor asthma symptoms data and also record and send medication according to the symptoms. Another important feature is that it records its data and sends it to the Google database.[74–76]

But certain parts of the body haven't been successfully scrutinized using cell phone-based attachments. Blood samples are one of them. Many important biomarkers such as vitamins, minerals, viruses, and cancer symptoms are measured from blood.

Except glucose, most of these biomarkers work at large amount of the sample. Their level are too low that they cannot be measured in a drop of blood.

It may one day be possible for people to check their blood samples on a routine basis using their cell phones to monitor their cancer or heart disease biomarker levels against baseline. Another possibility is that before having a relationship/intercourse, one may ask for a cell-phone-based HIV test.[77–85]

## 2.9 ADVANTAGES OF ARTIFICIAL INTELLIGENCE

### 2.9.1 Expanded healthcare access

AI plays a very important role in reducing or eliminating misdiagnosis, mishandling, or wrong treatments. Developing and underdeveloped nations have a lack of clinical doctors and trainees; therefore, such nations can apply the treatment and diagnosis based on AI algorithms.

### 2.9.2 Improves record-keeping

Electronic health records (EHRs) make the storing and management of medical treatment and diagnosis records easier. Voice recognition AI technology and dictation also improve the record-maintaining process.

### 2.9.3 Advanced immunotherapy

In cancer treatment, AI plays an important role. As there is no cure for cancer, immunotherapy is being used in the medication process. However, it is not applied to all patients as it is suitable for some patients only. So, immunotherapy patients can be easily identified by AI.[86–93]

## 2.10 AI CAPABILITIES, TRANSLATIONS, SUMMARIZATION, AND PREDICTION[94]

Table 2.1 summarizes the potential roles and capabilities of AI in various clinical scenarios.

## 2.11 RISK OF AI TOOLS

The following harms and risks may be possible due to AI:

- Patient harm due to AI errors
- Misuse of medical AI tools
- Bias in AI and the perpetuation of existing inequities
- Lack of transparency
- Privacy and security issues
- Gaps in accountability
- Obstacles in implementation

These risks can be minimized by the following steps:

- Human agency and oversight
- Technical robustness and safety
- Privacy and data governance
- Transparency
- Diversity, non-discrimination, and fairness
- Environmental and societal well-being
- Accountability

*Table 2.1* Potential role of AI and capacity of AI for clinical scenario

| *AI capability* | *Description* | *Example for clinical scenario* | *Potential role of AI* |
|---|---|---|---|
| Identification | Identifying objects, patterns, and/or characteristics within data (often images | A physician orders an X-ray for a patient who presents with pain, swelling, and limited leg mobility | An AI tool reviews the X-ray and identifies an incidental nodule for further analysis by a radiologist |
| Translation | Translating data inputs into another data type or data format (often between modalities or languages), often using natural language processing | A radiologist reviews an MRI for a patient at risk of breast cancer and dictates observations via an audio recording | An AI tool converts the radiologist's audio dictation into a structured summary and applies the BIRADS classification scheme automatically. The AI produces a "plain language" interpretation for the patient. The AI could also translate the report into a different language |
| Summarization | Summarizing data inputs into shorter and more accessible outputs | A patient is admitted to an emergency department in status epilepticus. A team of admitting healthcare professionals reviews the patient's medical file to understand the patient's medical history, current medications, previous allergic reactions, and potential triggering factors | An AI tool reviews the patient's medical history in totality, near instantly identifying and summarizing key information for current clinical needs, such as recent medication changes affecting seizure threshold, and a list of contraindicated drugs based on allergy history |
| Prediction | Predicting or forecasting future events based on historical data and patterns | A patient is discharged after hospitalization for heart failure. A patient is discharged after hospitalization for heart failure | Using historic heart failure readmission rates and the patient's clinical data, an AI tool predicts the risk of the patient's hospital readmission |

(*Continued*)

*Table 2.1* (Continued) Potential role of AI and capacity of AI for clinical scenario

| *AI capability* | *Description* | *Example for clinical scenario* | *Potential role of AI* |
|---|---|---|---|
| Suggestion | Providing recommendations, guidance, or advice. In some systems, suggestions may automatically lead to a specific downstream action | A patient sees a provider every few months for a routine check-in; the clinical team conducts a retrospective analysis of blood glucose measures from the past few months | An AI tool continually monitors a patient's blood glucose levels and (1) sends an alert to the patient and clinician when deviations occur and (2) provides a recommended course of action (e.g., insulin level recommendation) |

## 2.12 CONCLUSIONS

AI-based tools paired with advanced data science are increasing the sensitivity and the accuracy of clinical diagnosis and treatment. To develop effective AI systems, additional knowledge and data are essential to eliminate disease, conflict, and misery. Healthcare executives should consider ethical access to delicate, inconsistent, and compartmentalized healthcare data, domain expertise, and computational capacity for real-time decision-making. Cloud computing is transforming computational power, and research on its implementation is critical to ensuring that "trusted" AI algorithms are integrated into acceptable workflows. AI adoption and implementation in healthcare systems confront significant obstacles, including data quality, access, technological infrastructure, organizational capability, ethical principles, safety, and legislation. Not only should the benefits of the AI tools be kept in mind, but their potential risk factors should also be considered when using them. Risk factors can be minimized by the following seven types of steps: (1) human agency and oversight; (2) technical robustness and safety; (3) privacy and data governance; (4) transparency; (5) diversity, non-discrimination, and fairness; (6) environmental and societal well-being; and (7) accountability.

## LIST OF ABBREVIATIONS

| | |
|---|---|
| AAL | ambient-assisted living |
| AI | artificial intelligence |
| CDSS | clinical decision support system |
| DL | deep learning |
| DNN | deep neural network |
| DT | decision tree |

| | |
|---|---|
| EHR | electronic health record |
| GRU | Gated Recurrent Unit |
| HLA-DR | human leukocyte antigen-DR |
| KNN | k-nearest neighbor |
| LSTM | long short-term memory |
| ML | machine learning |
| MLBD | machine learning-based diagnosis |
| NLP | natural language processing |
| QSAR | quantitative structure–activity relationship |
| RF | random forest |
| SARS | severe acute respiratory syndrome |
| SMILES | simplified molecular input line entry system |
| SVM | support vector machine |
| UCI | University of California |

## CONFLICTS OF INTEREST

The authors declare no conflict of interest.

Diagrams were created with BioRender.com.

## REFERENCES

1. Paz, B. J., & Kai-Fu Lee (2019). AI superpowers—China, Silicon Valley and the new world order. *AI & Society*, 35(3), 771–772 (2020). https://doi.org/10.1007/s00146-019-00906-7
2. Holden, C. (1991). Machines who think. *Science*, 254(5036), 1608–1609.
3. Huang, L. F. (2010). Artificial intelligence. In *Proceedings of the 2nd international conference on computer and automation engineering (ICCAE 2010)* (Vol. 4). IEEE.
4. Hoyt, R. E., Snider, D., Thompson, C., & Mantravadi, S. (2016). IBM Watson analytics: Automating visualization, descriptive, and predictive statistics. *JMIR Public Health and Surveillance*, 2(2), e157. https://doi.org/10.2196/publichealth.5810
5. Show, M. B. H. (2018). *How AI is used in healthcare—5 powerful real-world examples and the latest advances*. Forbes.
6. Singhal, S., & Carlton, S. (2019). *The era of exponential improvement in healthcare?* McKinsey & Company.
7. Minaee, S., Kafieh, R., Sonka, M., Yazdani, S., & Jamalipour Soufi, G. (2020). Deep-COVID: Predicting COVID-19 from chest X-ray images using deep transfer learning. *Medical Image Analysis*, 65, 101794. https://doi.org/10.1016/j.media.2020.101794
8. Ahsan, M. M., Luna, S. A., & Siddique, Z. (2022). Machine-learning-based disease diagnosis: A comprehensive review. *Healthcare*, 10(1), 1–30. https://doi.org/10.3390/healthcare10010030

9. Ansari, A. Q., & Gupta, N. K. (2011). Automated diagnosis of coronary heart disease using neuro-fuzzy integrated system. In *Proceedings of the 2011 world congress on information and communication technologies (WICT 2011)* (pp. 1379–1384). IEEE. https://doi.org/10.1109/WICT.2011.6141450
10. Ahsan, M. M., Mahmud, M. A. P., Saha, P. K., Gupta, K. D., & Siddique, Z. (2021). Effect of data scaling methods on machine learning algorithms and model performance. *Technologies*, 9(3), 52. https://doi.org/10.3390/technologies9030052
11. Rubin, J., et al. (2017). Recognizing abnormal heart sounds using deep learning. *CEUR Workshop Proceedings*, 1891, 13–19.
12. Ahsan, M. M., & Siddique, Z. (2022). Machine learning-based heart disease diagnosis: A systematic literature review. *Artificial Intelligence in Medicine*, 128, 102276. https://doi.org/10.1016/j.artmed.2022.102276
13. World Health Organization. (2016). *Global report on diabetes*. World Health Organization. https://www.who.int/publications/i/item/9789241565257
14. Sarwar, N., et al. (2010). Diabetes mellitus, fasting blood glucose concentration, and risk of vascular disease: A collaborative meta-analysis of 102 prospective studies. *The Lancet*, 375(9733), 2215–2222. https://doi.org/10.1016/S0140-6736(10)60484-9
15. Kandhasamy, J. P., & Balamurali, S. (2015). Performance analysis of classifier models to predict diabetes mellitus. *Procedia Computer Science*, 47, 45–51. https://doi.org/10.1016/j.procs.2015.03.182
16. Varol, A., & Institute of Electrical and Electronics Engineers. (2020). *1st International informatics and software engineering conference (IISEC-2019): Innovative technologies for digital transformation*. IEEE.
17. Naz, H., & Ahuja, S. (2020). Deep learning approach for diabetes prediction using PIMA Indian dataset. *Journal of Diabetes & Metabolic Disorders*, 19, 391–403. https://doi.org/10.1007/s40200-020-00520-8
18. Ashiquzzaman, A., et al. (2017). Reduction of overfitting in diabetes prediction using deep learning neural network. In *Lecture notes in electrical engineering* (Vol. 449, pp. 35–43). Springer. https://doi.org/10.1007/978-981-10-3920-1_4
19. Alhassan, Z., et al. (2018). Type-2 diabetes mellitus diagnosis from time series clinical data using deep learning models. In *Lecture notes in computer science* (Vol. 11141, pp. 468–478). Springer. https://doi.org/10.1007/978-3-030-01331-1_42
20. Chan, J. F.-W., et al. (2020). A familial cluster of pneumonia associated with the 2019 novel coronavirus indicating person-to-person transmission: A study of a family cluster. *The Lancet*, 395(10223), 514–523. https://doi.org/10.1016/S0140-6736(20)30154-9
21. Mughees, M., Chugh, H., Naqvi, S. H., & Wajid, S. (2021). COVID-19 threat to the world: Current and possible diagnostic/treatment strategies. *Critical Reviews in Biomedical Engineering*, 49(1), 21–33. https://doi.org/10.1615/CritRevBiomedEng.2021037924
22. Chatterjee, S., Mishra, S., Chowdhury, K. D., Ghosh, C. K., & Saha, K. D. (2021). Various theranostics and immunization strategies based on nanotechnology against COVID-19 pandemic: An interdisciplinary view. *Life Sciences*, 278, 119580. https://doi.org/10.1016/j.lfs.2021.119580

23. Quek, E., Tahir, H., Kumar, P., Hastings, R., & Jha, R. (2021). Treatment of COVID-19: A review of current and prospective pharmacotherapies. *British Journal of Hospital Medicine*, 82(2), 1–8. https://doi.org/10.12968/hmed.2020.0615
24. Hamamoto, R., Suemizu, H., Nakamura, Y., & Furukawa, T. (2020). Application of artificial intelligence technology in oncology: Towards the establishment of precision medicine. *Cancers (Basel)*, 12(12), 3532. https://doi.org/10.3390/cancers12123532
25. Oh, Y., Park, S., & Ye, J. C. (2020). Deep learning COVID-19 features on CXR using limited training data sets. *IEEE Transactions on Medical Imaging*, 39(8), 2688–2700. https://doi.org/10.1109/TMI.2020.2993291
26. Kulkarni, A. R., et al. (2021). Deep learning model to predict the need for mechanical ventilation using chest X-ray images in hospitalised patients with COVID-19. *BMJ Innovations*, 7(2), 261–270. https://doi.org/10.1136/bmjinnov-2020-000611
27. Zandehshahvar, M., et al. (2021). Toward understanding COVID-19 pneumonia: A deep-learning-based approach for severity analysis and monitoring the disease. *Scientific Reports*, 11, 9570. https://doi.org/10.1038/s41598-021-88910-0
28. Chen, B., et al. (2019). Predicting HLA class II antigen presentation through integrated deep learning. *Nature Biotechnology*, 37(11), 1332–1343. https://doi.org/10.1038/s41587-019-0280-2
29. Morris, A., et al. (2021). Discovery of SARS-CoV-2 main protease inhibitors using a synthesis-directed de novo design model. *Chemical Communications*, 57(47), 5909–5912. https://doi.org/10.1039/D1CC01759B
30. Ke, Y.-Y., et al. (2020). Artificial intelligence approach fighting COVID-19 with repurposing drugs. *Biomedical Journal*, 43(4), 355–362. https://doi.org/10.1016/j.bj.2020.05.001
31. Lee, A. (2023). *Open science discovery of potent non-covalent SARS-CoV-2 main protease inhibitors* (pp. 1–31). https://doi.org/10.26434/chemrxiv-2023
32. Asada, K., et al. (2021). Application of artificial intelligence in COVID-19 diagnosis and therapeutics. *Journal of Personalized Medicine*, 11(9), 886. https://doi.org/10.3390/jpm11090886
33. Calzolari, D., et al. (2008). Search algorithms as a framework for the optimization of drug combinations. *PLoS Computational Biology*, 4(12), e1000249. https://doi.org/10.1371/journal.pcbi.1000249
34. Day, D., & Siu, L. L. (2016). Approaches to modernize the combination drug development paradigm. *Genome Medicine*, 8, 115. https://doi.org/10.1186/s13073-016-0362-7
35. Gupta, R., et al. (2021). Artificial intelligence to deep learning: Machine intelligence approach for drug discovery. *Molecular Diversity*, 25(3), 1317–1350. https://doi.org/10.1007/s11030-020-10168-6
36. Zhang, Y., et al. (2019). Construction of a targeting nanoparticle of 3′,3″-bis-peptide-siRNA conjugate/mixed lipid with postinserted DSPE-PEG2000-cRGD. *Molecular Pharmaceutics*, 16(11), 4920–4928. https://doi.org/10.1021/acs.molpharmaceut.9b00767

37. He, S., et al. (2019). Herb-induced liver injury: Phylogenetic relationship, structure–toxicity relationship, and herb–ingredient network analysis. *International Journal of Molecular Sciences*, 20(2), 363. https://doi.org/10.3390/ijms20020363
38. Zhang, D.-H., Wu, K.-L., Zhang, X., Deng, S.-Q., & Peng, B. (2020). In silico screening of Chinese herbal medicines with the potential to directly inhibit 2019 novel coronavirus. *Journal of Integrative Medicine*, 18(2), 152–158. https://doi.org/10.1016/j.joim.2020.02.005
39. National Research Council. (2011). *Toward precision medicine: Building a knowledge network for biomedical research and a new taxonomy of disease*. National Academies Press. https://doi.org/10.17226/13284
40. van der Schee, M., Pinheiro, H., & Gaude, E. (2018). Breath biopsy for early detection and precision medicine in cancer. *Ecancermedicalscience*, 12, 856. https://doi.org/10.3332/ecancer.2018.856
41. Hartmaier, R. J., Albacker, L. A., Chmielecki, J., Bailey, M., He, J., Goldberg, M. E., ... Frampton, G. M. (2017). High-throughput genomic profiling of adult solid tumors reveals novel insights into cancer pathogenesis. *Cancer Research*, 77(9), 2464–2475. https://doi.org/10.1158/0008-5472.CAN-16-2472
42. Piwek, L., Ellis, D. A., Andrews, S., & Joinson, A. (2016). The rise of consumer health wearables: Promises and barriers. *PLoS Medicine*, 13(2), e1001953. https://doi.org/10.1371/journal.pmed.1001953
43. Coravos, A., Khozin, S., & Mandl, K. D. (2019). Developing and adopting safe and effective digital biomarkers to improve patient outcomes. *NPJ Digital Medicine*, 2, 14. https://doi.org/10.1038/s41746-019-0090-4
44. Gold, M., Amatniek, J., Carrillo, M. C., Cedarbaum, J. M., Hendrix, J. A., Miller, B. B., ... Czaja, S. J. (2018). Digital technologies as biomarkers, clinical outcomes assessment, and recruitment tools in Alzheimer's disease clinical trials. *Alzheimer's & Dementia: Translational Research & Clinical Interventions*, 4, 234–242. https://doi.org/10.1016/j.trci.2018.04.003
45. Kim, T. H., Kim, D., Choi, J., Kim, B. W., Park, J., Kim, D. E., ... Lee, H. (2019). A temporary indwelling intravascular aphaeretic system for in vivo enrichment of circulating tumor cells. *Nature Communications*, 10, 1478. https://doi.org/10.1038/s41467-019-09493-6
46. Wernli, K. J., Henrikson, N. B., Morrison, C. C., Nguyen, M., Pocobelli, G., & Blasi, P. R. (2016). Screening for skin cancer in adults: Updated evidence report and systematic review for the US Preventive Services Task Force. *JAMA*, 316(4), 436–447. https://doi.org/10.1001/jama.2016.5415
47. Esteva, A., Kuprel, B., Novoa, R. A., Ko, J., Swetter, S. M., Blau, H. M., & Thrun, S. (2017). Dermatologist-level classification of skin cancer with deep neural networks. *Nature*, 542(7639), 115–118. https://doi.org/10.1038/nature21056
48. Abu-Hassan, K., Taylor, J. D., Morris, P. G., ... Heath, J. R. (2019). Optimal solid-state neurons. *Nature Communications*, 10(1), 5309. https://doi.org/10.1038/s41467-019-13374-w
49. Ahmed, Z., Mohamed, K., Zeeshan, S., & Dong, X. (2020). Artificial intelligence with multi-functional machine learning platform development for better healthcare and precision medicine. *Database: The Journal of Biological Databases and Curation, 2020*, baaa010. https://doi.org/10.1093/database/baaa010

50. Albarqouni, S., Baur, C., Achilles, F., Belagiannis, V., Demirci, S., & Navab, N. (2016). AggNet: Deep learning from crowds for mitosis detection in breast cancer histology images. *IEEE Transactions on Medical Imaging*, 35(5), 1313–1321. https://doi.org/10.1109/TMI.2016.2528120
51. Almada, M., & Maranhão, J. (2021). Voice-based diagnosis of COVID-19: Ethical and legal challenges. *International Data Privacy Law*, 11(2), ipab004. https://doi.org/10.1093/idpl/ipab004
52. Ameer, F., Singh, A. K., & Kumar, S. (2013). Evolution of instruments for harvest of skin grafts. *Indian Journal of Plastic Surgery*, 46(1), 28–35. https://doi.org/10.4103/0970-0358.113706
53. Astrakas, L. G., Naqvi, S. H., Kateb, B., & Tzika, A. A. (2012). Functional MRI using robotic MRI-compatible devices for monitoring rehabilitation from chronic stroke in the molecular medicine era (Review). *International Journal of Molecular Medicine*, 29(6), 963–973. https://doi.org/10.3892/ijmm.2012.934
54. Bali, J., Garg, R., & Bali, R. T. (2019). Artificial intelligence (AI) in healthcare and biomedical research: Why a strong computational/AI bioethics framework is required? *Indian Journal of Ophthalmology*, 67(1), 3–6. https://doi.org/10.4103/ijo.IJO_1627_18
55. Almada, M., & Maranhão, J. (2021). Voice-based diagnosis of COVID-19: Ethical and legal challenges. *International Data Privacy Law*, 11(2), ipab004. https://doi.org/10.1093/idpl/ipab004
56. Ameer, F., Singh, A. K., & Kumar, S. (2013). Evolution of instruments for harvest of skin grafts. *Indian Journal of Plastic Surgery*, 46(1), 28–35. https://doi.org/10.4103/0970-0358.113706
57. Astrakas, L. G., Naqvi, S. H., Kateb, B., & Tzika, A. A. (2012). Functional MRI using robotic MRI-compatible devices for monitoring rehabilitation from chronic stroke in the molecular medicine era (Review). *International Journal of Molecular Medicine*, 29(6), 963–973. https://doi.org/10.3892/ijmm.2012.934
58. Bali, J., Garg, R., & Bali, R. T. (2019). Artificial intelligence (AI) in healthcare and biomedical research: Why a strong computational/AI bioethics framework is required? *Indian Journal of Ophthalmology*, 67(1), 3–6. https://doi.org/10.4103/ijo.IJO_1627_18
59. Gillinov, A. M., Mihaljevic, T., Javadikasgari, H., Suri, R. M., Mick, S. L., Navia, J. L., ... Sabik, J. F. (2018). Early results of robotically assisted mitral valve surgery: Analysis of the first 1000 cases. *The Journal of Thoracic and Cardiovascular Surgery*, 155(1), 82–91. https://doi.org/10.1016/j.jtcvs.2017.08.099
60. Gouda, W., & Yasin, R. (2020). COVID-19 disease: CT pneumonia analysis prototype by using artificial intelligence, predicting the disease severity. *The Egyptian Journal of Radiology and Nuclear Medicine*, 51(1), 196. https://doi.org/10.1186/s43055-020-00291-9
61. Krittanawong, C., Zhang, H., Wang, Z., Aydar, M., & Kitai, T. (2017). Artificial intelligence in precision cardiovascular medicine. *Journal of the American College of Cardiology*, 69(21), 2657–2664. https://doi.org/10.1016/j.jacc.2017.03.571
62. Lanfranco, A. R., Castellanos, A. E., Desai, J. P., & Meyers, W. C. (2004). Robotic surgery: A current perspective. *Annals of Surgery*, 239(1), 14–21. https://doi.org/10.1097/01.sla.0000103020.19595.7d

63. Lang, J. E., Mannava, S., Floyd, A. J., Goddard, M. S., Smith, B. P., Mofidi, A., ... Seyler, T. M. (2011). Robotic systems in orthopaedic surgery. *The Journal of Bone and Joint Surgery*, 93(10), 1296–1299. https://doi.org/10.2106/JBJS.J.00723
64. Lee, H., Mittal, A., Patel, K., Gatuz, J. L., Truong, L., Torres, J., ... Chiang, C. M. (2014). Identification of novel drug scaffolds for inhibition of SARS-CoV 3-chymotrypsin-like protease using virtual and high-throughput screenings. *Bioorganic & Medicinal Chemistry*, 22(1), 167–177. https://doi.org/10.1016/j.bmc.2013.11.007
65. Almada, M., & Maranhão, J. (2021). Voice-based diagnosis of COVID-19: Ethical and legal challenges. *International Data Privacy Law*, 11(2), ipab004. https://doi.org/10.1093/idpl/ipab004
66. Nørgaard, B. L., Leipsic, J., Gaur, S., Seneviratne, S., Ko, B. S., Ito, H., ... Lassen, J. F. (2014). Diagnostic performance of noninvasive fractional flow reserve derived from coronary computed tomography angiography in suspected coronary artery disease: The NXT trial. *Journal of the American College of Cardiology*, 63(12), 1145–1155. https://doi.org/10.1016/j.jacc.2013.11.043
67. Taylor, C. A., Fonte, T. A., & Min, J. K. (2013). Computational fluid dynamics applied to cardiac computed tomography for noninvasive quantification of fractional flow reserve. *Journal of the American College of Cardiology*, 61(22), 2233–2241. https://doi.org/10.1016/j.jacc.2012.11.083
68. U.S. Food and Drug Administration. (2017, July). *FDA announces new steps to empower consumers and advance digital healthcare.* FDA Voice. https://blogs.fda.gov/fdavoice/index.php/2017/07/fda-announces-new-steps-to-empower-consumers-and-advance-digital-healthcare
69. International Medical Device Regulators Forum (IMDRF). (n.d.). *Software as a medical device (SaMD): Work items.* http://www.imdrf.org/workitems/wi-samd.asp
70. International Medical Device Regulators Forum (IMDRF). (2014). *Software as a medical device: Possible framework for risk categorization and corresponding considerations.* http://www.imdrf.org/docs/imdrf/final/technical/imdrf-tech-140918-samd-framework-risk-categorization-141013.pdf
71. International Medical Device Regulators Forum (IMDRF). (n.d.). *Software as a medical device: Clinical evaluation.* http://www.imdrf.org/docs/imdrf/final/consultations/imdrf-cons-samd-ce.pdf
72. U.S. Food and Drug Administration. (2016, October 14). *Software as a medical device (SaMD): Clinical evaluation—International Medical Device Regulators Forum (IMDRF) draft guidance. Federal Register.* https://www.federalregister.gov/documents/2016/10/14/2016-24805/software-as-a-medical-device- clinical-evaluation-international-medical-device-regulators-forum-draft
73. U.S. Food and Drug Administration. (n.d.). *Software as a medical device (SaMD).* FDA Voice. https://blogs.fda.gov/fdavoice/index.php/tag/software-as-a-medical-device-samd
74. AsthmaMD. (n.d.). *AsthmaMD.* http://www.asthmamd.org/
75. National Institutes of Health. (2017). *RFA-AG-18-012: Mobile monitoring of cognitive change (U2C/U54).* https://grants.nih.gov/grants/guide/rfa-files/RFA-AG-18-012.html

76. Doerr, M., Maguire Truong, A., Bot, B. M., Wilbanks, J., Suver, C., Mangravite, L. M., ... Kellen, M. (2017). Formative evaluation of participant experience with mobile eConsent in the app-mediated Parkinson mPower study: A mixed methods study. *JMIR mHealth and uHealth*, 5(2), e14. https://doi.org/10.2196/mhealth.6521
77. Peterson, K., Deeduvanu, R., Kanjamala, P., & Boles, K. (2016). *A blockchain-based approach to health information exchange networks*. Office of the National Coordinator for Health Information Technology. https://www.healthit.gov/sites/default/files/12-55-blockchain-based-approach-final.pdf
78. Health Level Seven International (HL7). (n.d.). *FHIR: Fast healthcare interoperability resources*. https://www.hl7.org/fhir/
79. Kaput, J., & Rodriguez, R. L. (2004). Nutritional genomics: The next frontier in the postgenomic era. *Physiological Genomics*, 16(2), 166–177. https://doi.org/10.1152/physiolgenomics.00107.2003
80. Vineis, P., & Wild, C. P. (2014). Global cancer patterns: Causes and prevention. *The Lancet*, 383(9916), 549–557. https://doi.org/10.1016/S0140-6736(13)62224-2
81. Landrigan, P. J., Lambertini, L., & Birnbaum, L. S. (2012). A research strategy to discover the environmental causes of autism and neurodevelopmental disabilities. *Environmental Health Perspectives*, 120(7), a258–a260. https://doi.org/10.1289/ehp.1104285
82. Volk, H. E., Hertz-Picciotto, I., Delwiche, L., Lurmann, F., & McConnell, R. (2011). Residential proximity to freeways and autism in the CHARGE study. *Environmental Health Perspectives*, 119(6), 873–877. https://doi.org/10.1289/ehp.1002835
83. Castorina, R., Butt, C., Stapleton, H. M., Avery, D., Harley, K. G., Holland, N., ... Bradman, A. (2017). Flame retardants and their metabolites in the homes and urine of pregnant women residing in California (the CHAMACOS cohort). *Chemosphere*, 179, 159–166. https://doi.org/10.1016/j.chemosphere.2017.03.076
84. Gulshan, V., Peng, L., Coram, M., Stumpe, M. C., Wu, D., Narayanaswamy, A., ... Webster, D. R. (2016). Development and validation of a deep learning algorithm for detection of diabetic retinopathy in retinal fundus photographs. *JAMA*, 316(22), 2402–2410. https://doi.org/10.1001/jama.2016.17216
85. Esteva, A., Kuprel, B., Novoa, R. A., Ko, J., Swetter, S. M., Blau, H. M., & Thrun, S. (2017). Dermatologist-level classification of skin cancer with deep neural networks. *Nature*, 542(7639), 115–118. https://doi.org/10.1038/nature21056
86. Kourou, K., Exarchos, K. P., Papaloukas, C., Sakaloglou, P., Exarchos, T., & Fotiadis, D. I. (2021). Applied machine learning in cancer research: A systematic review for patient diagnosis, classification, and prognosis. *Computational and Structural Biotechnology Journal*, 19, 5546–5555. https://doi.org/10.1016/j.csbj.2021.10.006
87. Price, W. N., & Cohen, I. G. (2019). Privacy in the age of medical big data. *Nature Medicine*, 25(1), 37–43. https://doi.org/10.1038/s41591-018-0272-7
88. Reddy, S., Fox, J., & Purohit, M. P. (2018). Artificial intelligence–enabled healthcare delivery. *Journal of the Royal Society of Medicine*, 112(1), 22–28. https://doi.org/10.1177/0141076818815510

89. Amann, J., Blasimme, A., Vayena, E., Frey, D., & Madai, V. I. (2020). Explainability for artificial intelligence in healthcare: A multidisciplinary perspective. *BMC Medical Informatics and Decision Making*, 20(1), 310. https://doi.org/10.1186/s12911-020-01332-6
90. Arnold, M. H. (2021). Teasing out artificial intelligence in medicine: An ethical critique of artificial intelligence and machine learning in medicine. *Journal of Bioethical Inquiry*, 18(1), 121–139. https://doi.org/10.1007/s11673-020-10080-1
91. Davenport, T., & Kalakota, R. (2019). The potential for artificial intelligence in healthcare. *Future Healthcare Journal*, 6(2), 94–98. https://doi.org/10.7861/futurehosp.6-2-94
92. Guan, J. (2019). Artificial intelligence in healthcare and medicine: Promises, ethical challenges, and governance. *Chinese Medical Sciences Journal*, 34(2), 99–107. https://doi.org/10.24920/003611
93. Khanna, D. (2020). Use of artificial intelligence in healthcare and medicine. *Open Science Framework (OSF Preprints)*. https://doi.org/10.31221/osf.io/eshm9
94. American Medical Association. (2021). *Future of health: Augmented intelligence in health care*. https://www.ama-assn.org/system/files/future-health-augmented-intelligence-health-care.pdf

Chapter 3

# Artificial intelligence in the treatment and diagnosis of infectious diseases

*Mohmmad Younus Wani*

## 3.1 INTRODUCTION

Infectious diseases continue to be a major global health threat, leading to millions of deaths and widespread morbidity annually [1]. Despite progress in medical interventions such as vaccines, treatments, and diagnostic tools, the burden of infectious diseases remains significant [2]. Pathogens, including bacteria, viruses, fungi, and parasites, are constantly evolving, often outstripping the effectiveness of current medical strategies aimed at preventing or treating infections. The rise of antimicrobial resistance (AMR), the rapid mutation of viruses like influenza and HIV, and the emergence of new and re-emerging infectious diseases emphasize the critical need for innovative solutions [3, 4].

Traditional methods for managing infectious diseases, such as microbiological testing, clinical assessment, and the use of broad-spectrum antibiotics, are increasingly insufficient in addressing these evolving challenges [5]. There is a growing demand for novel approaches that can not only facilitate faster detection and diagnosis of infectious diseases but also enable the customization of treatment plans, predict outbreaks, and accelerate the development of new antimicrobial agents. In this context, artificial intelligence (AI) has emerged as a transformative force with the potential to revolutionize the diagnosis, treatment, and management of infectious diseases [6–8].

AI encompasses a wide range of techniques, including machine learning (ML), deep learning (DL), natural language processing (NLP), and big data analytics, all of which can be leveraged in innovative ways within healthcare [6]. By processing vast amounts of data, including medical images, genetic sequences, patient histories, and epidemiological trends, AI has the potential to improve diagnostic accuracy, identify previously unrecognized patterns, and support more targeted treatment strategies [6, 7]. Furthermore, AI can assist in predicting disease outbreaks, monitoring the evolution of pathogens, and accelerating the discovery of new drugs and vaccines [9].

The integration of AI into healthcare marks a significant shift, offering the potential for faster, more accurate, and personalized care, particularly in low-resource settings where the burden of infectious diseases is most

DOI: 10.1201/9781003741770-3

pronounced [10]. This chapter will explore the expanding role of AI in the management of infectious diseases, focusing on its applications in diagnostic imaging, genetic sequencing, personalized treatment plans, and epidemiological modeling. We will also examine the ways in which AI is streamlining drug discovery and predicting the emergence of new pathogens, all while shaping the future landscape of global infectious disease management. However, the implementation of AI also presents challenges, including concerns around data privacy, algorithmic bias, and the need for comprehensive regulatory frameworks to ensure its safe and effective use.

## 3.2 AI IN INFECTIOUS DISEASE DIAGNOSIS

Accurate and timely diagnosis is critical for the effective treatment and management of infectious diseases, as well as for controlling their spread within populations [11]. Early detection enables healthcare providers to administer the appropriate treatment swiftly, mitigate the transmission of infectious agents, and prevent complications, particularly in vulnerable groups. However, traditional diagnostic methods such as culture-based techniques, polymerase chain reaction (PCR), and serological tests have notable limitations. These challenges include prolonged turnaround times, high costs, reliance on specialized laboratory infrastructure, and issues with sensitivity and specificity, especially when detecting novel or emerging pathogens. To address these challenges, artificial intelligence (AI) has emerged as a promising solution to transform the diagnostic landscape (Table 3.1). AI technologies, notably machine learning (ML) and deep learning (DL), have the potential to enhance traditional diagnostic techniques by providing quicker, more accurate, and cost-efficient identification of infectious diseases. By streamlining diagnostic workflows, improving data interpretation, and delivering real-time results, AI can significantly support rapid decision-making in clinical settings and public health interventions.

### 3.2.1 AI for diagnostic imaging

Medical imaging represents one of the most impactful areas where AI has enhanced the diagnosis of infectious diseases [12]. Deep learning techniques, especially convolutional neural networks (CNNs), have shown exceptional capability in analyzing imaging data from modalities like X-rays, CT scans, MRIs, and ultrasounds. These algorithms can be trained to detect subtle patterns indicative of infections in various organs, including the lungs and brain. For example, AI-powered systems have been used to examine chest X-rays and identify conditions such as pneumonia, tuberculosis, and COVID-19-related lung abnormalities. In the context of COVID-19, AI has been particularly effective in recognizing patterns of viral pneumonia, such

*Table 3.1* AI applications in infectious disease diagnosis

| *AI application area* | *Description* | *Benefits* | *Examples* |
|---|---|---|---|
| AI for diagnostic imaging | AI, particularly deep learning (DL) models like convolutional neural networks (CNNs), analyzes medical images (X-rays, CT scans, MRIs) to identify patterns linked to infections. | Faster, more accurate diagnosis<br>Reduces reliance on expert radiologists<br>Cost-effective | Chest X-rays for pneumonia, tuberculosis, and COVID-19<br>MRI and CT scans for detecting infections in organs |
| AI for microbial identification | AI, combined with next-generation sequencing (NGS), processes genomic data to identify pathogens, mutations, and resistance markers. | Rapid identification of pathogens<br>Improved detection of emerging strains<br>Shortens diagnosis timeline | Genomic analysis for bacterial, viral, and fungal infections<br>AI analysis of NGS data to track mutations in pathogens like COVID-19 and influenza |
| AI for point-of-care diagnostics | Portable diagnostic devices using AI algorithms to analyze samples at the site of care, such as blood smears, using smartphone cameras and sensors. | Quick, accessible diagnosis<br>Low cost<br>Can be used in resource-limited settings | Malaria detection via smartphone images<br>AI-driven mobile apps for tuberculosis, HIV, or bacterial infection diagnosis |
| AI for syndromic diagnosis | AI processes complex patient data (symptoms, medical history, environment) to predict possible infectious diseases, aiding clinicians in making faster decisions. | Supports rapid diagnosis when specific pathogens are difficult to identify<br>More informed clinical decisions | AI models predicting conditions like influenza, COVID-19, and bacterial pneumonia based on symptoms such as fever, cough, and fatigue |
| AI for predictive diagnostics | AI models predict the likelihood of developing specific infectious diseases based on risk factors and historical data, guiding preventive measures and early interventions. | Proactive disease management<br>Tailored interventions for high-risk individuals | Risk prediction models for tuberculosis, HIV, and hepatitis<br>Predicting outbreaks of infectious diseases based on historical and environmental data |

as ground-glass opacities and consolidation, often seen on chest imaging [13]. These AI systems have demonstrated diagnostic accuracy that rivals, or even surpasses, that of human radiologists, providing a valuable solution to the shortage of skilled medical professionals, particularly in resource-limited areas.

AI is also being utilized in the detection of other infectious diseases, such as malaria, through the analysis of blood smear images [14]. Deep learning models can accurately distinguish between infected and non-infected cells in blood samples, offering quicker and more precise diagnostic results compared to traditional manual microscopy, which is time-consuming and prone to human error.

### 3.2.2 AI for microbial identification

AI is also revolutionizing the field of microbial identification, providing significant improvements over traditional methods [15]. Conventional techniques, such as culture-based methods, require isolating and cultivating pathogens in the lab, a process that can take several days or even weeks. By integrating AI with advanced sequencing technologies, the time required for microbial detection can be drastically reduced, and the accuracy of identification is enhanced.

Next-generation sequencing (NGS) technologies, which enable the rapid and high-throughput sequencing of pathogen genomes, are particularly advantageous for diagnosing infections caused by novel or rare microorganisms [16]. AI models are capable of processing the vast amounts of genomic data produced by NGS, allowing for the swift identification of microbial species, tracking of genetic variations, and detection of resistance markers. By analyzing large datasets from well-characterized pathogens, AI can also detect new mutations or emerging strains of known infectious agents, facilitating early intervention in outbreak scenarios.

Furthermore, AI-driven natural language processing (NLP) systems can mine literature databases, scientific publications, and clinical records to help identify potential causative agents in cases where the infection remains unidentified by traditional methods [17]. These AI tools can cross-reference clinical symptoms, geographic data, and patient outcomes to propose likely pathogens, thus supporting clinicians in making more informed decisions when faced with diagnostic challenges.

### 3.2.3 AI for point-of-care diagnostics

In many regions, especially low- and middle-income countries, access to advanced diagnostic laboratories is often limited, and patients may need to travel long distances to receive care. AI offers a promising solution to bridge this gap by enabling point-of-care (POC) diagnostics, where diagnostic tools are deployed directly at the site of patient care [18]. These tools typically incorporate portable sensors, smartphone cameras, and AI algorithms to analyze samples and deliver instant diagnostic results. For instance, AI-powered mobile applications can analyze images of blood samples to detect malaria parasites, identify bacterial infections, or assess the presence of other diseases, such as tuberculosis or HIV. In certain instances, these systems utilize the built-in cameras of smartphones to capture high-resolution images, which are then processed by AI algorithms to identify abnormalities or pathogens.

Point-of-care AI diagnostic devices offer numerous advantages, including faster result turnaround, lower costs, and the ability to function in resource-constrained settings [18]. These tools can be used by healthcare workers who may not have specialized training in advanced diagnostic methods, empowering them to make informed decisions directly at the patient's location and reducing the workload on overwhelmed central laboratories.

### 3.2.4 AI for syndromic diagnosis

In many instances, infectious diseases manifest with a variety of nonspecific symptoms, making it challenging to determine the exact causative agent. Syndromic diagnosis, which involves identifying diseases based on symptom patterns rather than specific pathogens, is a method that can be significantly enhanced by AI [19]. AI systems are capable of processing diverse data, including patient medical histories, symptom profiles, demographic details, and even environmental factors, to identify potential infections and suggest the most probable causes. Machine learning algorithms can be trained to analyze these complex and multifactorial datasets, helping clinicians quickly narrow down the differential diagnosis. For example, a patient presenting with fever, cough, and fatigue could have several potential diagnoses, such as influenza, COVID-19, or bacterial pneumonia. AI-powered decision support systems can integrate available data to prioritize the most likely diagnoses, enabling clinicians to select appropriate diagnostic tests and initiate treatment more promptly.

### 3.2.5 AI for predictive diagnostics and risk assessment

AI models are also being leveraged to predict the likelihood of a patient developing a specific infectious disease based on individual risk factors [20]. These predictive tools use historical patient data, epidemiological trends, and other relevant variables to forecast disease progression, aiding in the implementation of preventive measures. For instance, AI algorithms can evaluate the risk of infection in patients with underlying conditions, such as immunocompromised individuals, and suggest personalized preventive strategies or early interventions. These predictive models are especially valuable in managing diseases like tuberculosis, HIV, or hepatitis, where early detection and timely intervention can greatly improve long-term outcomes.

Moreover, AI can enhance public health surveillance by predicting the occurrence of infectious disease outbreaks [6]. By analyzing historical data and environmental factors, including climate change, human migration, and population density, AI models can anticipate potential outbreaks, enabling public health authorities to initiate timely interventions and mitigate widespread transmission.

## 3.3 AI IN INFECTIOUS DISEASE TREATMENT

The treatment of infectious diseases is a dynamic and often intricate process, involving the selection of the most suitable therapeutic agents based on the pathogen, the patient's clinical condition, and the potential for drug resistance [21]. While traditional treatment methods have proven effective in numerous instances, challenges such as antimicrobial resistance (AMR), the emergence of novel pathogens, and the variability in individual patient responses have made it increasingly difficult to manage infectious diseases effectively. Artificial intelligence (AI) holds significant promise in enhancing the treatment of infectious diseases by improving drug discovery, optimizing treatment protocols, predicting patient responses, and facilitating personalized medicine. These advancements could lead to better treatment outcomes, reduced adverse effects, and a more efficient approach to managing both existing and emerging infectious threats.

### 3.3.1 AI for drug discovery

The development of new antimicrobial drugs, including antibiotics, antivirals, antifungals, and antiparasitic agents, is essential to combat the growing threat of resistant pathogens [21]. However, traditional drug discovery methods are time-consuming and expensive and often fail to yield effective treatments. AI has emerged as a transformative tool in drug discovery, offering the ability to accelerate the identification of promising compounds, predict their efficacy, and optimize their properties [22].

Machine learning (ML) and deep learning (DL) algorithms can analyze large datasets of molecular structures, biological activities, and clinical trial outcomes to identify potential drug candidates more efficiently and accurately than traditional methods. AI can simulate the interaction between drugs and pathogens at the molecular level, predicting how well specific molecules will bind to target proteins involved in the infectious disease process. This helps identify novel compounds that could serve as effective therapeutics.

One significant advantage of AI in drug discovery is its potential to repurpose existing drugs for new uses [23]. By analyzing data from clinical trials, patient outcomes, and molecular databases, AI algorithms can uncover existing medications that may be effective against emerging infectious diseases. For example, during the COVID-19 pandemic, AI played a crucial role in screening existing drugs for potential efficacy against the novel coronavirus, leading to the identification of repurposed treatments such as remdesivir and dexamethasone. Additionally, AI can assist in identifying new drug-resistant mechanisms, supporting the design of drugs targeting these newly discovered resistance pathways. In this way, AI can help address the growing challenge of antimicrobial resistance by facilitating the development of more effective drugs, whether novel or repurposed.

### 3.3.2 AI for treatment optimization

AI has the potential to significantly enhance the optimization of treatment regimens for patients with infectious diseases [6]. The primary goal of treatment optimization is to ensure that patients receive the most effective medication at the appropriate dosage, tailored to their unique characteristics and the specific nature of their infection. This is particularly critical in infectious diseases like HIV, tuberculosis, and hepatitis, where long-term therapy is often required. Optimizing treatment regimens in these cases is essential for improving patient outcomes and reducing the risk of resistance.

Machine learning algorithms can analyze patient-specific data, including medical history, demographic factors, genetic information, and microbiological results, to predict the most effective treatment plans [24]. For instance, AI models can incorporate factors such as a patient's genetic profile, their ability to metabolize specific drugs, the presence of co-infections, and the likelihood of resistance to certain medications, allowing for personalized treatment recommendations. In the case of HIV, AI can assess the viral load, resistance profile, and previous treatment history of the patient's virus to predict the most effective combination of antiretroviral drugs [25]. This approach not only boosts treatment efficacy but also reduces the risk of developing drug resistance, which is a major concern in chronic infections.

Similarly, for tuberculosis (TB), AI can predict the likelihood of drug resistance based on genetic data from *Mycobacterium tuberculosis*, assisting clinicians in selecting the appropriate first- or second-line drugs. This capability is especially important given the increasing prevalence of multidrug-resistant (MDR) and extensively drug-resistant (XDR) tuberculosis strains. Additionally, AI can optimize dosing schedules by incorporating real-time data from wearable devices, such as blood pressure monitors, glucose meters, or pulse oximeters. Continuous monitoring allows AI to adjust treatment regimens dynamically, ensuring that patients always receive the most appropriate care. This ability to make real-time treatment adjustments helps minimize side effects, avoid drug interactions, and improve overall patient outcomes.

### 3.3.3 AI for personalized medicine in infectious diseases

Personalized medicine, which customizes medical treatment to the unique characteristics of each patient, is gaining prominence in the treatment of infectious diseases [26]. Rather than relying on a one-size-fits-all approach, personalized medicine enables clinicians to factor in a patient's genetic profile, microbiome, immune response, and other relevant factors to offer more precise and effective treatment.

AI can significantly enhance personalized medicine in the context of infectious disease treatment by analyzing extensive, multidimensional datasets to predict how a particular patient will respond to specific treatments [27]. By integrating genetic, proteomic, and metabolomic data, AI models can identify biomarkers that forecast how a patient will metabolize a drug, the likelihood of side effects, or the risk of treatment failure. For example, AI can identify genetic variations in patients that affect the metabolism of drugs like antimalarials or antibiotics, allowing for more accurate dosing and reducing the risk of adverse reactions.

Beyond genetic factors, AI can also analyze the microbiome, which plays a crucial role in a patient's susceptibility to infections and their response to treatment. The human microbiome can impact the efficacy of numerous drugs, including antibiotics, and AI algorithms can identify which microbial populations are present in the patient's system. This information can guide more targeted therapies by ensuring that the chosen drugs do not disrupt beneficial microbial communities and help clinicians select treatments more likely to be effective. Understanding how the microbiome influences treatment outcomes and resistance mechanisms can help clinicians choose therapies with the best chance of success.

AI-driven personalized treatment plans extend beyond just drug selection and dosing. These systems can also predict the patient's recovery trajectory, identify potential complications, and enable more effective follow-up care. For instance, AI can predict which patients are at high risk of adverse events, such as sepsis or organ failure, allowing for early intervention and more intensive monitoring when necessary.

## 3.4 AI IN MANAGING ANTIMICROBIAL RESISTANCE (AMR)

Antimicrobial resistance (AMR) has emerged as a critical global health concern, significantly complicating the treatment of various infectious diseases

[28]. The rise of drug-resistant pathogens—whether bacterial, viral, fungal, or parasitic—leads to increased treatment failures, longer hospital stays, and higher mortality rates. AI offers a powerful means to tackle the multifaceted challenge of AMR by enhancing our ability to detect, monitor, and respond to emerging resistance trends [29].

Advanced AI algorithms can process vast genomic datasets from clinical and environmental sources to identify resistance-associated mutations and track their evolution over time. This capability allows for early detection of resistance patterns, helping clinicians and public health authorities anticipate shifts in pathogen behavior and adjust treatment protocols accordingly. By pinpointing genetic markers linked to resistance, AI can predict which strains are at risk of developing resistance to specific antimicrobials, supporting more proactive and informed decision-making. Furthermore, AI can aid in antimicrobial stewardship by improving the precision of antibiotic usage. Machine learning models can assess infection severity, patient characteristics, and microbial profiles to recommend appropriate antibiotic types and durations. This personalized guidance helps reduce the overuse and misuse of antimicrobials—key drivers of resistance. For example, AI tools can support decisions about when to discontinue antibiotics safely, thus limiting unnecessary exposure and preserving the effectiveness of current treatments.

## 3.5 AI IN INFECTIOUS DISEASE SURVEILLANCE AND GLOBAL HEALTH

Artificial intelligence (AI) has become an indispensable tool for strengthening global health infrastructure, particularly in the surveillance and control of infectious diseases [30, 31]. By harnessing AI-driven predictive models, health systems can monitor the emergence and spread of infectious agents in real time. These technologies analyze diverse datasets, including epidemiological records, environmental variables, climate trends, and human travel patterns to anticipate where and when outbreaks may occur. Such predictive insights are critical for preemptive action. AI can help identify potential outbreak hotspots and populations at risk, allowing public health agencies to deploy targeted interventions more efficiently. This includes directing resources such as vaccines, diagnostic kits, and healthcare personnel to areas with the highest projected disease burden. In outbreaks involving pathogens like influenza, malaria, or Ebola, early forecasting facilitated by AI can significantly reduce transmission rates and improve containment strategies.

By integrating large-scale data from multiple sources, AI not only enhances the accuracy of surveillance but also contributes to a more agile and responsive global health system, capable of adapting quickly to emerging threats and minimizing the impact of infectious disease crises.

## 3.6 AI IN EPIDEMIOLOGY AND OUTBREAK PREDICTION

Epidemiology plays a central role in understanding the dynamics of disease transmission and shaping effective public health responses [31]. While traditional epidemiological approaches rely on data reported by healthcare systems, laboratories, and governmental bodies, they are often hampered by delays, incomplete information, and the overwhelming volume of data required to monitor rapidly evolving outbreaks. Artificial intelligence (AI) offers a transformative advantage by processing extensive, heterogeneous datasets—including electronic health records (EHRs), global health surveillance reports, environmental data, and even social media activity—to detect patterns and anomalies indicative of emerging health threats [32].

By integrating machine learning (ML) and deep learning (DL) techniques, AI models can identify early warning signals of disease outbreaks, model transmission dynamics, and forecast the geographic spread of infections with improved precision. These tools are capable of updating in real time, allowing for adaptive modeling that reflects current trends and changing epidemiological conditions.

AI-driven epidemiological surveillance systems significantly enhance the speed and accuracy of outbreak detection and response. They allow public health authorities to act more decisively by providing timely insights into where an outbreak may occur next, which populations are at greatest risk, and how interventions might curb transmission. This is especially critical for managing high-impact infectious diseases, such as those caused by novel viruses or pathogens with pandemic potential, where rapid containment can save lives and prevent widespread disruption.

### 3.6.1 Predicting disease outbreaks

Artificial intelligence (AI) has emerged as a valuable tool in forecasting infectious disease outbreaks before they escalate into major public health crises [30]. By examining a combination of variables such as transmission dynamics, weather patterns, travel data, and human behavioral trends, AI models can anticipate when and where an outbreak may occur—often earlier than traditional surveillance systems can detect.

These predictive capabilities allow for more proactive public health responses. Authorities can act swiftly by deploying vaccines, medical supplies, or health personnel to high-risk areas, helping to contain the spread of infection. This early-warning approach not only improves the efficiency of outbreak management but also reduces the overall burden on healthcare systems and affected communities.

#### *3.6.1.1 Machine learning algorithms for outbreak prediction*

Machine learning (ML) plays a pivotal role in predicting disease outbreaks by enabling the analysis of highly complex and evolving datasets [33]. These algorithms can process vast amounts of historical and real-time data—such as epidemiological records, demographic profiles, environmental variables, and socio-economic indicators—to detect subtle trends that might signal the onset of an outbreak. For example, ML models can identify early warnings of recurring diseases like seasonal influenza by examining spikes in symptoms, patterns in healthcare utilization, and regional anomalies in disease reporting. This early detection gives health systems crucial time to prepare for an influx of patients.

In the case of emerging or less predictable infectious threats such as Ebola, Zika, or COVID-19, ML algorithms are capable of synthesizing inputs from diverse sources—including environmental data (e.g., rainfall, temperature), local surveillance reports, and global travel networks—to estimate the likelihood and location of potential outbreaks. These data-driven forecasts help guide health officials in prioritizing at-risk regions and deploying preventive interventions to contain the spread.

#### *3.6.1.2 Geospatial analysis and climate conditions*

Artificial intelligence (AI) models increasingly incorporate geospatial data to monitor and anticipate the spread of infectious diseases across regions [34]. By integrating Geographic Information Systems (GIS) with AI, researchers can generate dynamic risk maps that visually represent areas most susceptible to disease outbreaks. These tools allow for real-time tracking and modeling of disease propagation based on geographic and population-based variables.

Climate factors, such as temperature, humidity, and rainfall, play a vital role in influencing the spread of many infectious diseases, particularly those transmitted by vectors like mosquitoes. For instance, vector-borne illnesses such as malaria, dengue, and Zika are closely linked to environmental conditions that support mosquito breeding and survival. AI systems can analyze long-term climate data and establish correlations with historical outbreak patterns to forecast regions at elevated risk. This is particularly important in tropical and subtropical areas where seasonal climate changes can significantly alter disease dynamics, enabling targeted surveillance and timely public health responses.

### 3.6.2 Modeling disease spread and predicting healthcare burden

Following the detection of an outbreak, artificial intelligence (AI) can play a key role in forecasting how an infectious disease may spread and in estimating the impact it will have on healthcare systems [35]. By combining real-time data with advanced epidemiological modeling, AI can simulate various outbreak scenarios and predict how an infection might propagate across regions. These insights enable authorities to estimate future case numbers and anticipate pressure points in healthcare delivery.

AI-based models consider multiple variables—such as population density, travel behavior, intervention strategies, and public compliance with health guidelines—to predict how infections like COVID-19, tuberculosis, or influenza may evolve. Additionally, they can forecast healthcare demands, including hospital bed occupancy, ICU admissions, and the need for life-support equipment. This foresight supports better planning and resource distribution, helping hospitals and public health agencies prepare in advance and avoid being overwhelmed during critical phases of an outbreak.

## 3.7 CHALLENGES AND ETHICAL CONSIDERATIONS

Although artificial intelligence (AI) holds great promise in transforming how infectious diseases are diagnosed and treated, its application also introduces several technical and ethical hurdles that must be carefully managed, as summarized in Table 3.2. One major concern is safeguarding patient privacy, as AI depends on vast amounts of medical data, often containing confidential and personally identifiable information. Ensuring secure data handling, informed consent, and robust cybersecurity protocols is essential to protect patient rights.

Another key issue is the potential for bias in AI models. If training data lacks diversity or is skewed, the AI may produce unreliable or inequitable outcomes, potentially exacerbating existing health disparities. Additionally, inconsistencies or gaps in healthcare data can limit the effectiveness of AI systems, reducing their accuracy and reliability.

For AI to be trusted in clinical settings, its decision-making processes must be transparent and explainable. Healthcare professionals and patients must understand how AI reaches its conclusions, especially when those insights inform critical care decisions. Ethical concerns also arise regarding responsibility and accountability for AI-driven outcomes, equitable access to AI tools across different regions and populations, and maintaining a supportive rather than substitutive role for AI alongside human expertise.

To address these issues, a coordinated effort involving clinicians, data scientists, ethicists, and policymakers is essential. Such collaboration can

*Table 3.2* Challenges and ethical considerations in AI for infectious disease diagnosis

| *Challenge/ethical issue* | *Description* | *Impact* | *Solutions* |
|---|---|---|---|
| Data privacy and security | Concerns about patient consent, data protection, and cybersecurity. | Risk of data breaches and misuse | Implement encryption, GDPR/HIPAA compliance, and transparent consent mechanisms |
| Bias in AI algorithms | AI models may inherit biases from unrepresentative data, affecting diagnosis accuracy. | Inaccurate results, especially for underserved groups | Use diverse datasets and conduct regular fairness audits |
| Data quality and availability | Incomplete or fragmented healthcare data can hinder AI model accuracy. | Poor AI performance and limited generalization | Standardize data collection, foster collaboration, and improve data annotation |
| Algorithmic transparency | AI models' "black-box" nature can limit the interpretability of decisions. | Lack of trust and understanding among users | Develop explainable AI (XAI) models and increase transparency in decision-making processes |
| Ethical use and accountability | Clear accountability is needed for AI-driven errors or adverse outcomes. | Legal and ethical concerns over mistakes | Establish clear accountability guidelines and involve human oversight |
| Equitable access | Unequal access to AI technology, especially in low-resource settings. | Widening healthcare disparities | Develop affordable AI solutions and invest in infrastructure for broad access |

help ensure that AI technologies are implemented fairly, ethically, and to the benefit of all communities in infectious disease prevention and control.

## 3.8 FUTURE DIRECTIONS

The application of artificial intelligence (AI) in diagnosing and managing infectious diseases is poised for significant growth, driven by rapid advancements in machine learning, natural language processing, and data analytics. As these technologies mature, AI is expected to play an increasingly central role in transforming healthcare delivery, especially in regions with limited medical infrastructure. In the coming years, AI will contribute to more accurate, timely, and personalized healthcare solutions. Innovations such as AI-powered diagnostic tools, intelligent drug discovery platforms, and real-time outbreak prediction systems are expected to become more sophisticated and widely accessible. These developments will not only enhance clinical decision-making but also support public health responses to emerging disease threats.

Moreover, the integration of AI with other emerging fields, such as genomics, robotics, and telemedicine, will create powerful synergies, enabling more holistic and proactive approaches to infectious disease control. Continued interdisciplinary collaboration and investment in AI research will be essential to ensure that these technologies are implemented effectively and equitably across global healthcare systems.

## 3.9 CONCLUSION

Artificial intelligence is set to play a transformative role in reshaping the landscape of infectious disease diagnosis and treatment. By leveraging advanced technologies such as machine learning, deep learning, and big data analytics, AI has the potential to accelerate drug discovery, fine-tune treatment protocols, and enable faster, more precise diagnostics. Despite the challenges that still need to be addressed, the integration of AI into healthcare systems holds tremendous promise for improving global health management, offering a powerful tool to combat some of the most urgent infectious disease threats worldwide.

## REFERENCES

1. Bloom DE, Cadarette D. Infectious disease threats in the twenty-first century: strengthening the global response. *Front Immunol.* 2019;10:549. doi:10.3389/fimmu.2019.00549.
2. Baker RE, Mahmud AS, Miller IF, Rajeev M, Rasambainarivo F, Rice BL, et al. Infectious disease in an era of global change. *Nat Rev Microbiol.* 2022;20(4):193–205. doi:10.1038/s41579-021-00639-z.
3. Prestinaci F, Pezzotti P, Pantosti A. Antimicrobial resistance: a global multifaceted phenomenon. *Pathog Glob Health.* 2015;109(7):309–318. doi:10.1179/2047773215Y.0000000030.
4. Nii-Trebi NI. Emerging and neglected infectious diseases: insights, advances, and challenges. *Biomed Res Int.* 2017;2017:5245021. doi:10.1155/2017/5245021.
5. Yamin D, Uskoković V, Wakil AM, Goni MD, Shamsuddin SH, Mustafa FH, et al. Current and future technologies for the detection of antibiotic-resistant bacteria. *Diagnostics.* 2023;13(20):3246. doi:10.3390/diagnostics13203246.
6. Srivastava V, Kumar R, Wani MY, Robinson K, Ahmad A. Role of artificial intelligence in early diagnosis and treatment of infectious diseases. *Infect Dis.* 2024;1–26. doi:10.1080/23744235.2024.2425712.

7. Zhang X, Zhang D, Zhang X, Zhang X. Artificial intelligence applications in the diagnosis and treatment of bacterial infections. *Front Microbiol.* 2024;15:1449844. doi:10.3389/fmicb.2024.1449844.
8. Hirani R, Noruzi K, Khuram H, Hussaini AS, Aifuwa EI, Ely KE, et al. Artificial intelligence and healthcare: a journey through history, present innovations, and future possibilities. *Life.* 2024;14(5):557. doi:10.3390/life14050557.
9. Olawade DB, Teke J, Fapohunda O, Weerasinghe K, Usman SO, Ige AO, et al. Leveraging artificial intelligence in vaccine development: a narrative review. *J Microbiol Methods.* 2024;224:106998. doi:10.1016/j.mimet.2024.106998.
10. Zuhair V, Babar A, Ali R, Oduoye MO, Noor Z, Chris K, et al. Exploring the impact of artificial intelligence on global health and enhancing healthcare in developing nations. *J Prim Care Community Health.* 2024;15:21501319241245847. doi:10.1177/21501319241245847.
11. Mukherjee R, Vidic J, Auger S, Wen HC, Pandey RP, Chang CM. Exploring disease management and control through pathogen diagnostics and One Health initiative: a concise review. *Antibiotics (Basel).* 2023 Dec;13(1):17. doi:10.3390/antibiotics13010017.
12. Chu WT, Reza SMS, Anibal JT, Landa A, Crozier I, Bağci U, et al. Artificial intelligence and infectious disease imaging. *J Infect Dis.* 2023 Oct 3;228(Suppl 4):S322–S336. doi:10.1093/infdis/jiad158.
13. Nagpal P, Narayanasamy S, Vidholia A, Guo J, Shin KM, Lee CH, et al. Imaging of COVID-19 pneumonia: patterns, pathogenesis, and advances. *Br J Radiol.* 2020 Sep 1;93(1113):20200538. doi:10.1259/bjr.20200538.
14. Liu R, Liu T, Dan T, Yang S, Li Y, Luo B, et al. AIDMAN: an AI-based object detection system for malaria diagnosis from smartphone thin-blood-smear images. *Patterns (N Y).* 2023 Aug 3;4(9):100806. doi:10.1016/j.patter.2023.100806.
15. Shelke YP, Badge AK, Bankar NJ. Applications of artificial intelligence in microbial diagnosis. *Cureus.* 2023 Nov 24;15(11):e49366. doi:10.7759/cureus.49366.
16. Satam H, Joshi K, Mangrolia U, Waghoo S, Zaidi G, Rawool S, et al. Next-generation sequencing technology: current trends and advancements. *Biology (Basel).* 2023 Jul 13;12(7):997. doi:10.3390/biology12070997.
17. Al Kuwaiti A, Nazer K, Al-Reedy A, Al-Shehri S, Al-Muhanna A, Subbarayalu AV, et al. A review of the role of artificial intelligence in healthcare. *J Pers Med.* 2023 Jun 5;13(6):951. doi:10.3390/jpm13060951.
18. Khan AI, Khan M, Khan R. Artificial intelligence in point-of-care testing. *Ann Lab Med.* 2023 Sep 1;43(5):401–407. doi:10.3343/alm.2023.43.5.401.
19. Zhang X, Zhang D, Zhang X, Zhang X. Artificial intelligence applications in the diagnosis and treatment of bacterial infections. *Front Microbiol.* 2024 Aug 6;15:1449844. doi:10.3389/fmicb.2024.1449844.
20. Mayer LM, Strich JR, Kadri SS, Lionakis MS, Evans NG, Prevots DR, et al. Machine learning in infectious disease for risk factor identification and hypothesis generation: proof of concept using invasive candidiasis. *Open Forum Infect Dis.* 2022 Aug 3;9(8):ofac401. doi:10.1093/ofid/ofac401.
21. Muteeb G, Rehman MT, Shahwan M, Aatif M. Origin of antibiotics and antibiotic resistance, and their impacts on drug development: a narrative review. *Pharmaceuticals (Basel).* 2023 Nov 15;16(11):1615. doi:10.3390/ph16111615.

22. Visan AI, Negut I. Integrating artificial intelligence for drug discovery in the context of revolutionizing drug delivery. *Life (Basel)*. 2024 Feb 7;14(2):233. doi:10.3390/life14020233.
23. Vora LK, Gholap AD, Jetha K, Thakur RRS, Solanki HK, Chavda VP. Artificial intelligence in pharmaceutical technology and drug delivery design. *Pharmaceutics*. 2023 Jul 10;15(7):1916. doi:10.3390/pharmaceutics15071916.
24. Alowais SA, Alghamdi SS, Alsuhebany N, et al. Revolutionizing healthcare: the role of artificial intelligence in clinical practice. *BMC Med Educ*. 2023;23:689. doi:10.1186/s12909-023-04698-z.
25. Dixon D, Sattar H, Moros N, Kesireddy SR, Ahsan H, Lakkimsetti M, et al. Unveiling the influence of AI predictive analytics on patient outcomes: a comprehensive narrative review. *Cureus*. 2024 May 9;16(5):e59954. doi:10.7759/cureus.59954.
26. Goetz LH, Schork NJ. Personalized medicine: motivation, challenges, and progress. *Fertil Steril.* 2018 Jun;109(6):952–963. doi:10.1016/j.fertnstert.2018.05.006.
27. Johnson KB, Wei WQ, Weeraratne D, Frisse ME, Misulis K, Rhee K, et al. Precision medicine, AI, and the future of personalized health care. *Clin Transl Sci.* 2021 Jan;14(1):86–93. doi:10.1111/cts.12884.
28. Salam MA, Al-Amin MY, Salam MT, Pawar JS, Akhter N, Rabaan AA, et al. Antimicrobial resistance: a growing serious threat for global public health. *Healthcare (Basel)*. 2023 Jul 5;11(13):1946. doi:10.3390/healthcare11131946.
29. Branda F, Scarpa F. Implications of artificial intelligence in addressing antimicrobial resistance: innovations, global challenges, and healthcare's future. *Antibiotics (Basel)*. 2024 May 29;13(6):502. doi:10.3390/antibiotics13060502.
30. Sarantopoulos A, Mastori Kourmpani C, Yokarasa AL, Makamanzi C, Antoniou P, Spernovasilis N, et al. Artificial intelligence in infectious disease clinical practice: an overview of gaps, opportunities, and limitations. *Trop Med Infect Dis*. 2024;9(10):228. doi:10.3390/tropicalmed9100228.
31. Ryu S, Chun JY, Lee S, Yoo D, Kim Y, Ali ST, et al. Epidemiology and transmission dynamics of infectious diseases and control measures. *Viruses*. 2022 Nov 12;14(11):2510. doi:10.3390/v14112510.
32. Bajwa J, Munir U, Nori A, Williams B. Artificial intelligence in healthcare: transforming the practice of medicine. *Future Healthc J*. 2021 Jul;8(2):e188–e194. doi:10.7861/fhj.2021-0095.
33. Al Meslamani AZ, Sobrino I, de la Fuente J. Machine learning in infectious diseases: potential applications and limitations. *Ann Med.* 2024 Dec;56(1):2362869. doi:10.1080/07853890.2024.2362869.
34. Wang S, Huang X, Liu P, Zhang M, Biljecki F, Hu T, et al. Mapping the landscape and roadmap of geospatial artificial intelligence (GeoAI) in quantitative human geography: an extensive systematic review. *Int J Appl Earth Obs Geoinf.* 2024;128:103734. doi:10.1016/j.jag.2024.103734.
35. Varnosfaderani SM, Forouzanfar M. The role of AI in hospitals and clinics: transforming healthcare in the 21st century. *Bioengineering*. 2024;11(4):337. doi:10.3390/bioengineering11040337.

Chapter 4

# The role of artificial intelligence in diabetes

## A review of recent advances

*Mridul Sharma, Gaurav Kumar, Santosh Kumar, Shalinee Singh, Prem Anurag, and Imran Khan*

### 4.1 INTRODUCTION

Diabetes mellitus (DM) is a chronic metabolic disorder characterized by hyperglycemia due to defects in insulin secretion, insulin action, or both. It is a major cause of death globally and directly causes 1.6 million deaths annually. Type I, Type II, and gestational diabetes are the three main forms of diabetes, and the most prevalent is Type II, which accounts for almost 90% of all diabetes. Type I diabetes is an autoimmune condition that leads to the loss of insulin-secreting beta cells of the pancreas, while Type II is due to insulin resistance and relative insulin deficiency. Gestational diabetes is a pregnancy-related condition that is detrimental to both the mother and the child [1]. The manifestations of diabetes are widespread, involving multiple organs and leading to cardiovascular disease, nephropathy, neuropathy, and retinopathy. In 2017, the International Diabetes Federation (IDF) estimated that almost 8.8% of adults aged 20–79 years globally had diabetes, of whom half were unaware of the fact. The number of individuals with diabetes is estimated to be 439 million by 2030 and will rise to at least 592 million by 2035 [2]. The disease disproportionately affects men and is more common in urban than in rural areas. Traditional diabetes management includes lifestyle modification, glucose monitoring, and pharmacotherapy. These interventions, however, fail to prevent complications and attain optimal glycemic control.

Over the past few years, artificial intelligence (AI) has been a game-changer in diabetes management, promising early detection, risk prediction, personalized treatment, and complication management. AI and its subdisciplines, such as machine learning (ML) and deep learning (DL), enable the processing of large and intricate healthcare data, revealing patterns impossible for humans [3]. AI applications in diabetes management are diverse and illustrated in Figure 4.1. AI-based predictive models enable prediction of those at high risk of developing diabetes years before they develop it, facilitating timely interventions [4, 5]. For instance, AI-based algorithms can predict diabetes risk with high accuracy by analyzing electronic health records (EHRs), genetic information, and lifestyle factors. In diagnostics,

DOI: 10.1201/9781003741770-4

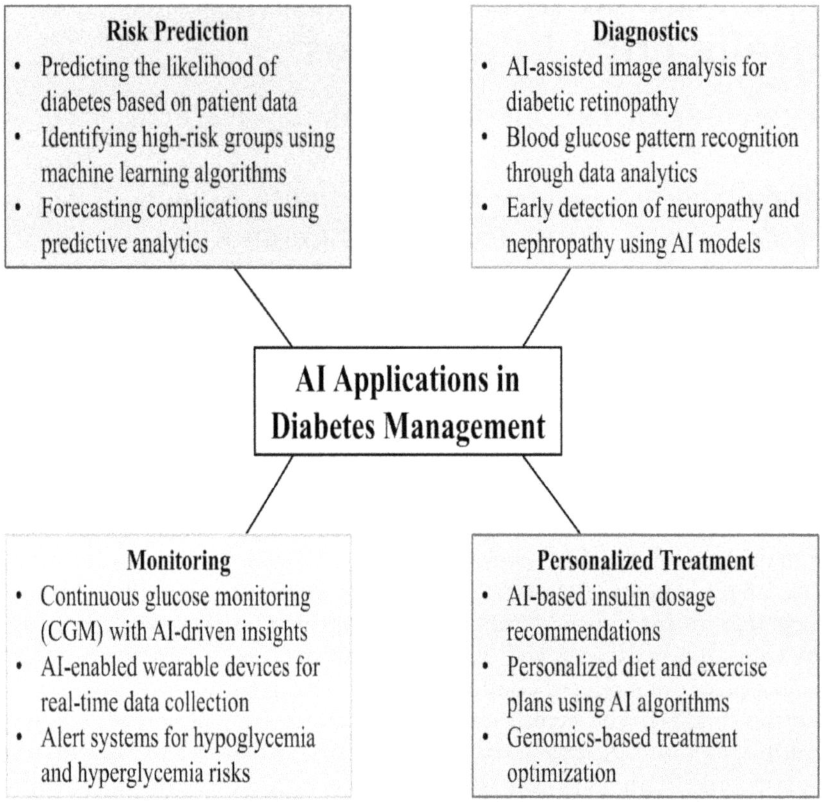


*Figure. 4.1* AI applications in diabetes management

AI-based image analysis has achieved success in the detection of diabetic retinopathy and other complications by identifying them through automated screening of retinal images, even outperforming experts. Moreover, AI can revolutionize personalized medicine by analyzing genetic profiles, metabolic information, and treatment response, advising clinicians on the best treatment regimen [6]. AI-based mobile health apps and wearables are also enabling patients to manage their condition proactively, giving real-time feedback on glucose levels, food intake, and physical activity. Despite its potential, the incorporation of AI in routine diabetes care is difficult, with obstacles such as data privacy issues, ethical concerns, and regulatory requirements. Overcoming these obstacles is essential for the large-scale application of AI-based solutions in diabetes care. Overall, AI promises revolutionary capabilities in diabetes care, ranging from risk prediction to personalized treatment, toward a proactive and accurate management of this global health challenge [7, 8].

This flowchart illustrates the various AI applications in diabetes management, including risk prediction, diagnostics, personalized treatment, and monitoring. Each segment highlights the specific roles of AI, such as predictive analytics, AI-assisted diagnostics, personalized therapy plans, and continuous monitoring systems.

## 4.2 AI IN DIABETIC RISK PREDICTION

Artificial intelligence has emerged as a powerful tool in diabetic risk prediction using large volumes of healthcare data, including electronic health records (EHRs), genetic information, lifestyle information, and continuous glucose monitoring information. Predictive models based on artificial intelligence can identify people who are likely to develop diabetes years in advance, allowing them to be treated early and preventive interventions to be initiated [4]. AI framework for diabetes management is illustrated in Figure 4.2.

Machine learning (ML) algorithms, as a branch of AI, are of supreme significance in predicting diabetic risk. Techniques such as support vector machines (SVMs), decision trees, and artificial neural networks (ANNs) have been found to be extremely precise in predicting the risk of diabetes on the basis of clinical parameters such as age, body mass index (BMI), blood pressure, and fasting glucose level [4]. Deep learning models have also been employed to screen retinal images in order to pick up early signs of diabetic retinopathy, which is typically an indicator of diabetes. Natural language processing (NLP) is another artificial intelligence technique that is gaining popularity to extract meaningful information from clinical notes and unstructured patient records. NLP programs are able to augment diabetic risk estimation by identifying patterns and relationships between these words [5].

The newer technologies include the integration of AI with mobile health apps and wearables. AI wearables monitor blood glucose continuously, activity, and vital signs and utilize the real-time data to predict hypoglycemic or hyperglycemic attacks. The real-time feedback mechanism not only facilitates the prediction of risk but also allows the patient to better control the disease [6]. In addition, predictive models based on AI have been shown to forecast the onset of Type II diabetes 5–10 years before clinical diagnosis, allowing a valuable window of opportunity for prevention by lifestyle intervention and early pharmacologic intervention [3]. AI's capacity to read across information sources and provide proper diabetic risk estimates makes it a game-changing tool in diabetes care. The combination of AI with real-time monitoring and personalized health advice holds tremendous potential to lower the global burden of diabetes.

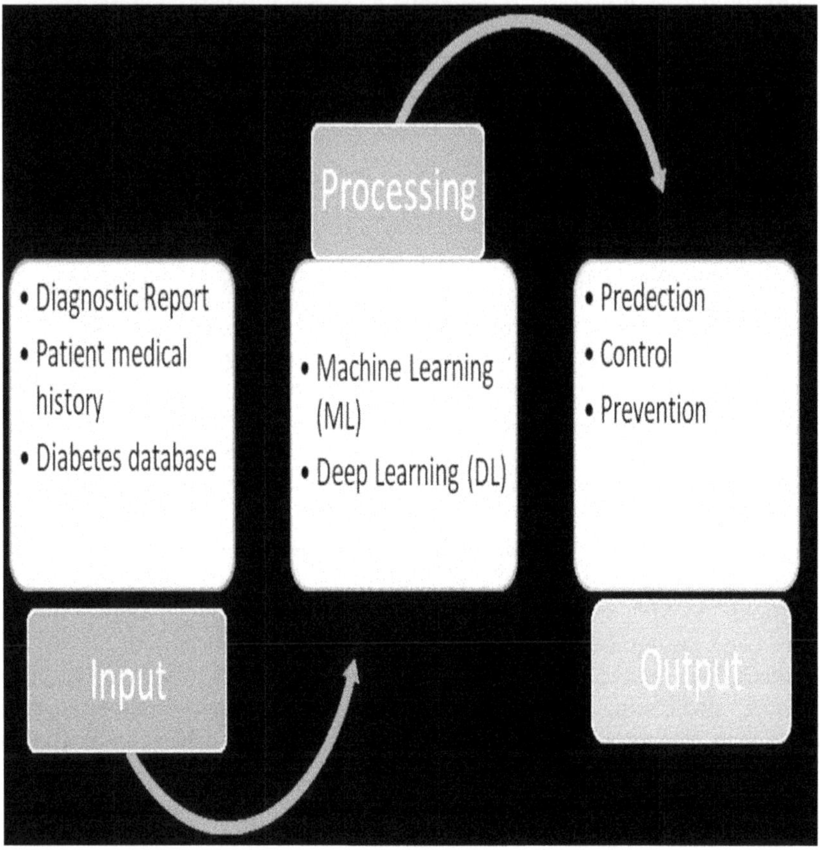


*Figure. 4.2* AI framework for diabetes management: The diagram illustrates the AI-based process of diabetes treatment starting with input (diabetes databases, patient's medical history, and diagnostic reports). The data are processed through machine learning (ML) and deep learning (DL) methods to generate output in the form of diabetes management prediction, control, and prevention measures

## 4.3 AI-ENABLED DIAGNOSTICS

Artificial intelligence (AI) diagnostics have transformed diabetes care through enhanced precision, efficiency, and speed of disease detection and monitoring. Through the use of machine learning (ML) algorithms and deep models, AI can analyze complex healthcare data, including imaging, laboratory, and clinical documentation, to identify patterns that are not necessarily apparent to human clinicians. One of the greatest advances in AI-based diagnostics has been the use of convolutional neural networks (CNNs) in medical imaging analysis. In diabetes, CNNs have been used to diagnose diabetic retinopathy (DR) with similar diagnostic accuracy as specialist ophthalmologists using computerized retinal fundus image analysis [3]. AI-based systems such as IDx-DR have even been approved by the Food and Drug Administration (FDA) for standalone diabetic retinopathy screening, ensuring the clinical applicability of AI-based diagnostics.

AI enhances diagnostic accuracy through natural language processing (NLP), which scans for relevant information in unstructured clinical text. Through the analysis of such texts, AI can identify early warning signs, diabetes complications, and comorbidities. AI algorithms based on recurrent neural networks (RNNs) and support vector machines (SVMs) have also been applied to electronic health records (EHRs) to forecast the risk of diabetes complications such as nephropathy and cardiovascular disease [5]. In clinical laboratory testing, point-of-care technology has been integrated with AI algorithms to assess glycated hemoglobin (HbA1c) levels, insulin sensitivity, and beta-cell function. Integration of these technologies facilitates rapid and precise assessments, allowing timely clinical decision-making. AI has also been used in continuous glucose monitoring (CGM) systems, where predictive algorithms forecast glucose fluctuations, allowing patients and healthcare providers to prepare for insulin dosing and food adjustment [6].

The ability of AI to access and process information from multiple sources also enables individualized diagnostic protocols. For instance, AI systems can combine genetic data, lifestyle parameters, and biomarker levels to categorize patients based on risk profiles and streamline diagnostic procedures with reduced or no unnecessary tests. Artificial intelligence diagnostics are a paradigm shift in diabetes management through accurate, personalized, and timely diagnostic tests that surpass conventional diagnosis. The continuous development of AI technology is expected to further improve diagnostic accuracy and patient outcomes in diabetes management.

## 4.4 AI TECHNIQUES IN DIABETES MANAGEMENT

Artificial intelligence methods have transformed diabetes care with the potential of accurate diagnosis, customized treatment, and ongoing monitoring. The primary AI methods used are supervised learning, unsupervised learning, reinforcement learning, deep learning, and hybrid AI models.

### 4.4.1 Supervised learning

Supervised learning involves training algorithms on labeled data to produce precise predictions of outcomes. In diabetes management, techniques such as decision trees, support vector machines (SVMs), and random forests have been employed to forecast the risk of diabetes and complications based on clinical parameters such as blood glucose levels, body mass index (BMI), and genetics [4]. SVM has been applied to forecast Type II diabetes based on demographic and lifestyle determinants with an over 85% accuracy rate. Artificial neural networks (ANNs) have been employed to forecast diabetic nephropathy risk from laboratory tests and vital signs [5].

### 4.4.2 Unsupervised learning

Unsupervised learning has been utilized for discovering intrinsic patterns in unlabeled data. K-means clustering and hierarchical clustering have been used to classify diabetes patients into subgroups based on risk profiles and drug response. Clustering algorithms have been used, for instance, to classify subtypes of Type II diabetes patients based on different metabolic and genetic features, to enable personalized therapy strategies [3].

### 4.4.3 Reinforcement learning

Reinforcement learning (RL) is directed toward decision-making optimization through learning from feedback. In diabetes care, RL algorithms have been employed in closed-loop insulin infusion systems, where they adjust insulin doses dynamically according to real-time glucose levels. For example, the use of deep Q-learning networks in artificial pancreas systems has been demonstrated to improve glycemic control and reduce hypoglycemic events [6].

### 4.4.4 Deep learning

Deep learning, a branch of machine learning, applies artificial neural networks of greater than one layer to learn large amounts of data. Convolutional neural networks (CNNs) have been used to identify diabetic retinopathy from retinal scans with diagnostic accuracy comparable to experienced ophthalmologists. Recurrent neural networks (RNNs) have been used in continuous glucose monitoring (CGM) data for glucose trend prediction and prevention of hyperglycemic and hypoglycemic events [5].

### 4.4.5 Hybrid AI models

Combining more than one AI method, hybrid models provide greater accuracy and stability in diabetes care. For example, combining supervised learning with reinforcement learning has been employed in the optimization of insulin dosing advice based on past and real-time information. Hybrid models combining CNNs and RNNs have also been employed in predicting diabetes complications from both image and time-series data, with more detailed risk predictions [3].

AI techniques provide an extensive array of tools for diabetes management, ranging from predicting the risk to specific treatment and online monitoring. Continuous development of AI techniques will keep pushing diabetes management progress ahead and demand interdisciplinary collaboration and ethical reflection.

## 4.5 PERSONALIZED TREATMENT AND MEDICATION OPTIMIZATION

Personalized diabetes treatment is focused on tailoring the treatment modalities according to the genetic profile, lifestyle, and clinical presentation of a person. AI is central to this since it utilizes big data to identify biomarkers, predict the outcomes of treatment, and propose individualized interventions.

### 4.5.1 Artificial intelligence in genetic profiling and biomarkers

AI software, particularly machine learning-based software, can analyze genetic data to establish risk loci for Type II diabetes and complications. For instance, AI has been used to analyze single-nucleotide polymorphisms (SNPs) to predict patient response to metformin, which is one of the most common diabetes medications. By identifying possibly responding patients to prescribed medications, AI helps alleviate side effects and optimize therapeutic outcomes [9].

### 4.5.2 Medication optimization

AI systems have been utilized to optimize insulin treatment in the management of diabetes. For instance, reinforcement learning algorithms have been incorporated into artificial pancreas systems to modify insulin delivery adaptively according to feedback from real-time glucose monitoring. AI systems also suggest dosage change for oral hypoglycemic drugs on the basis of trends in the pattern of blood glucose and drug compliance patterns [10].

### 4.5.3 Personalized lifestyle and nutrition counseling

Wearable devices and mobile health apps with AI capabilities can also provide personalized lifestyle and nutrition counseling to manage diabetes in the best possible way. AI algorithms, for instance, can analyze continuous glucose monitoring (CGM) data and suggest consumption frequency, portions, and exercise regimens that result in minimal glycemic fluctuation.

The apps not only maximize glycemic control but also enhance treatment adherence of patients [11].

### 4.5.4 Personalized treatment case studies

A case in point is the use of AI by Virta Health, a firm that employs machine learning algorithms to provide personalized ketogenic diet regimens to diabetic patients, resulting in dramatic reductions in HbA1c levels and insulin consumption. Another case in point is the use of AI by IBM Watson Health to recommend personalized medication regimens by integrating information from electronic health records (EHRs), genetic information, and lifestyle [12, 13].

The ability of AI to analyze heterogeneous sources of data offers a platform to transition from one-size-fits-all approaches to truly personalized diabetes management. With AI fine-tuning medications, dietary recommendations, and lifestyle modifications, therapeutic outcomes for diabetic patients are significantly enhanced.

## 4.6 AI FOR DIABETIC RETINOPATHY DETECTION

Diabetic retinopathy (DR) is a very serious diabetes-related complication that causes vision loss or blindness if it goes undetected. AI has come a long way in detecting diabetic retinopathy with accurate, effective, and scalable screening tools. Convolutional neural networks (CNNs) have been exceptionally successful in the classification of retinal fundus images to detect microaneurysms, hemorrhages, and exudates—early diabetic retinopathy indicators [5].

One of the most dramatic applications of AI here is Google's DeepMind, which developed an AI system that could diagnose over 50 eye diseases, including diabetic retinopathy, as accurately as specialist ophthalmologists. Another remarkable AI-driven solution is IDx-DR, which was approved by the FDA as the first autonomous AI diagnostic system for screening diabetic retinopathy without requiring an interpretation by a specialist. This solution uses a CNN-based algorithm to analyze an image from a retinal camera and output an immediate diagnosis, making it particularly valuable in primary care practice where access to ophthalmologists may be restricted [14].

Mobile AI-based apps are also transforming diabetic retinopathy screening. For instance, the EyeArt AI platform enables the autonomous screening of diabetic retinopathy using smartphone-enabled retinal cameras. The platform enhances access to screening services, especially in underserved and rural areas. AI programs that combine picture data and health history of a patient have, in addition, been developed in order to make predictions regarding developing diabetic retinopathy and personally tailored treatment planning, such as laser therapy or anti-VEGF injections [15]. The predictive analysis helps in facilitating early intervention along with the avoidance of disease acceleration [6].

The use of AI in the detection of diabetic retinopathy not only enhances the accuracy of diagnosis but also enables rapid and inexpensive screenings, lowering the risk of blindness in diabetes patients by a substantial amount.

## 4.7 AI FOR DIABETIC FOOT ULCER DETECTION

Diabetic foot ulcers (DFUs) are a serious diabetic complication that develops in approximately 15% of diabetic patients during their lifetime and frequently leads to infection, amputation, and serious morbidity. Early diagnosis and effective treatment of DFUs are crucial to prevent serious outcomes. AI has been identified as a potential tool in diabetic foot ulcer diagnosis and treatment through advanced image analysis, predictive modeling, and real-time monitoring [16].

### 4.7.1 AI-assisted image analysis

Convolutional neural networks (CNNs), being a type of deep learning models, have produced promising accuracy in the detection of DFU from smartphone- or digital-camera-captured images. For instance, CNN-driven systems are capable of differentiating among different grades of ulcer severity depending on depth, infection, and tissue type by scanning images of wounds. DeepConvNet is one such type, which was reported to be more than 90% accurate in identifying and classifying DFUs based on a labeled image database of wounds [17].

### 4.7.2 Predictive modeling of risk assessment

Predictive modeling entails the application of machine learning algorithms such as decision trees and support vector machines (SVMs) to forecast the risk of the development of DFUs from predictors such as blood glucose level, neuropathy status, and history of past wounds. The models assist clinicians in identifying early high-risk patients and instituting preventive interventions such as specialty footwear and regular foot check-ups [4, 18].

### 4.7.3 AI-based mobile applications

AI-based mobile applications such as FootSnap and PodoScanner enable patients to track foot health from the comfort of their homes. Since they can take and analyze photos of the feet, the apps provide instant feedback regarding the risk of ulceration and recommend follow-up actions, improving patient compliance and reducing the burden on the healthcare system [18, 19].

### 4.7.4 Integration with wearable sensors

AI-integrated wearable sensors can monitor pressure distribution, temperature differences, and gait patterns of diabetic patients in real time. AI algorithms process this data to identify anomalies indicating ulcer formation, enabling early interventions. As an example, AI-driven smart insoles can notify patients to offload pressure when abnormal stress is identified at specific regions of the foot [20].

Hence, the use of AI in diagnosing diabetic foot ulcers enhances the accuracy of diagnosis, enables proactive and targeted care, reduces amputations, and optimizes the quality of life in diabetic patients.

## 4.8 AI IN CONTINUOUS GLUCOSE MONITORING (CGM)

AI has greatly improved continuous glucose monitoring (CGM) systems by accurately forecasting glucose variability, thereby avoiding hypo- and hyperglycemic events. AI algorithms, especially recurrent neural networks (RNNs) and long short-term memory (LSTM) networks, are used to process CGM data and forecast glucose levels 60 minutes in advance. For example, the use of AI in CGM systems like the Medtronic Guardian Connect system has shown enhanced glycemic control by offering predictive prompts to patients. AI-based CGM systems also facilitate personalized insulin dosing by detecting patterns associated with meals, exercise, and stress, therefore improving the control of Type I diabetes [21].

## 4.9 ARTIFICIAL INTELLIGENCE IN PREVENTIVE DIABETES CARE

AI is also crucial in preventive diabetes management by detecting individuals at risk and suggesting timely interventions. Predictive analysis with AI can scan electronic health records (EHRs) to detect patterns that forecast the development of Type II diabetes. Support vector machine (SVM) and decision tree-based AI models, for instance, have been utilized to screen prediabetic patients on the basis of clinical and lifestyle information with accuracy levels of over 85%. AI-powered mobile apps such as BlueStar also utilize predictive algorithms to provide lifestyle suggestions, such as diet and exercise, designed to prevent diabetes development [22].

## 4.10 AI IN REMOTE DIABETES MANAGEMENT

The use of AI in remote diabetes care has revolutionized patient care by allowing continuous monitoring, telemedicine consultations, and real-time decision-making. Mobile apps like mySugr and Glooko, powered by AI, review data from CGM wearables and smart insulin pens to provide real-time, actionable feedback on insulin dosing and carbohydrate consumption. Natural language processing (NLP) combined with AI chatbots also helps patients by responding to diabetes-related questions and reminding them when to take medication. Additionally, AI-driven remote monitoring systems with predictive algorithms help healthcare professionals identify patients at risk of complications, allowing for timely interventions [23].

## 4.11 CHALLENGES AND ETHICAL CONSIDERATIONS

The application of AI in managing diabetes has significant benefits, but it has several challenges and ethical concerns that must be addressed to facilitate fair and ethical access. These are data privacy, algorithmic bias, regulatory compliance, and interpretability of AI models [10]. AI applications use vast quantities of individual health data, including electronic health records (EHRs), genotypic data, and real-time blood glucose monitoring data. Protection of such sensitive data against privacy and security breaches is of paramount importance. Compliance with regulations such as the Health Insurance Portability and Accountability Act (HIPAA) for the United States and the General Data Protection Regulation (GDPR) for the European Union must be followed to prevent data breaches and unauthorized access [5].

AI algorithms can perpetuate or even amplify biases in healthcare in an unintentional manner if trained on biased data. For instance, underrepresentation of certain demographic groups in training data can lead to less accurate predictions for the groups. Bias is tackled by careful dataset curation and use of fairness-aware machine learning to deliver equal healthcare to all patients with diabetes [24]. The pace of AI progress has surpassed the development of regulatory structures to guide its application in medicine. Standard guidelines for AI-based medical devices, such as standardization, validation, and approval processes, must be applied for safe use [25]. Institutions like the FDA have started addressing such issues by developing pathways for AI-assisted diagnostics, but there are loopholes in regulating predictive and personalized uses of AI [26]. AI models, especially deep learning models, are criticized as "black boxes" with outputs that are hard to explain. Failure to explain AI decisions erodes trust between patients and healthcare providers, hence the low uptake of AI-based solutions. Developing interpretable AI models capable of providing good explanations of their predictions is crucial in establishing trust and ensuring accountability [27]. Overcoming these issues and ethical challenges is essential for the safe integration of AI in diabetes care. A proper balance between innovation and ethical requirements will allow AI to achieve its full potential for the revolutionization of diabetes care.

## 4.12 CONCLUSION

The incorporation of artificial intelligence (AI) in the treatment of diabetes is a transformation from the conventional method of care to a personalized, proactive, and precise approach. AI, in its capacity to interpret large healthcare data, enables early risk prediction, precise diagnosis, tailored treatment regimens, and effective management of diabetes-related complications, including diabetic retinopathy and foot ulcers. Through the application of machine learning algorithms, deep learning models, and hybrid AI systems, clinicians can make evidence-based decisions that have a considerable impact on improving patient outcomes. Though promising much, AI-based management of diabetes is marred by several issues including privacy concerns with data, algorithmic bias, regulatory issues, and AI decision-making explainability. Addressing these issues with robust ethical standards and regulatory structures is key to establishing trust and promoting fair access to AI-supported healthcare interventions. With the advancement of AI technologies, it will be important for healthcare professionals, data scientists, and policymakers to collaborate across disciplines to make the best use of the full potential of AI in diabetes care. The future of diabetes care lies in the effective integration of technically robust and ethically robust AI systems to result in a more efficient, patient-centered model of managing this global health problem. Lastly, AI has distinct potential to revolutionize diabetes treatment with higher predictive power, better diagnosis, and customized treatment,, resulting in lower global burden of diabetes.

## REFERENCES

1. R. Khan, Z. Chua, J. Tan, Y. Yang, Z. Liao, and Y. Zhao, "From pre-diabetes to diabetes: diagnosis, treatments and translational research," *Medicina (B. Aires)*., vol. 55, no. 9, p. 546, Aug. 2019, doi: 10.3390/medicina55090546.
2. "International Diabetes Federation," IDF Diabetes Atlas, 10th edn. Brussels, Belgium, 2021. https://diabetesatlas.org/.
3. V. Buch, G. Varughese, and M. Maruthappu, "Artificial intelligence in diabetes care," *Diabet. Med.*, vol. 35, no. 4, pp. 495–497, Apr. 2018, doi: 10.1111/dme.13587.

4. A. Mujumdar and V. Vaidehi, "Diabetes prediction using machine learning algorithms," *Procedia Comput. Sci.*, vol. 165, pp. 292–299, 2019, doi: 10.1016/j.procs.2020.01.047.
5. J. Chaki, S. Thillai Ganesh, S. . Cidham and S. Ananda Theertan, "Machine learning and artificial intelligence based diabetes mellitus detection and self-management: a systematic review," *J. King Saud Univ. Comput. Inf. Sci.*, vol. 34, no. 6, pp. 3204–3225, Jun. 2022, doi: 10.1016/j.jksuci.2020.06.013.
6. I. Dankwa-Mullan, M. Rivo, M. Sepulveda, Y. Park, J. Snowdon, and K. Rhee, "Transforming diabetes care through artificial intelligence: the future is here," *Popul. Health Manag.*, vol. 22, no. 3, pp. 229–242, Jun. 2019, doi: 10.1089/pop.2018.0129.
7. C. D. Collins *et al.*, "The application of genomic and proteomic technologies in predictive, preventive and personalized medicine," *Vascul. Pharmacol.*, vol. 45, no. 5, pp. 258–267, Nov. 2006, doi: 10.1016/j.vph.2006.08.003.
8. P. Pesl *et al.*, "Case-based reasoning for insulin bolus advice," *J. Diabetes Sci. Technol.*, vol. 11, no. 1, pp. 37–42, Jan. 2017, doi: 10.1177/1932296816629986.
9. M. Jabara *et al.*, "Artificial intelligence-based digital biomarkers for type 2 diabetes: a review," *Can. J. Cardiol.*, vol. 40, no. 10, pp. 1922–1933, Oct. 2024, doi: 10.1016/j.cjca.2024.07.028.
10. Z. Guan *et al.*, "Artificial intelligence in diabetes management: advancements, opportunities, and challenges," *Cell Reports Med.*, vol. 4, no. 10, p. 101213, Oct. 2023, doi: 10.1016/j.xcrm.2023.101213.
11. S. Kannenberg *et al.*, "Unlocking potential: personalized lifestyle therapy for type 2 diabetes through a predictive algorithm-driven digital therapeutic," *J. Diabetes Sci. Technol.*, Jul. 2024, doi: 10.1177/19322968241266821.
12. Z. He and W. Li, "AI-driven management of type 2 diabetes in china: opportunities and challenges," *Diabetes, Metab. Syndr. Obes.*, vol. Volume 18, pp. 85–92, Jan. 2025, doi: 10.2147/DMSO.S495364.
13. S. J. Hallberg *et al.*, "Effectiveness and safety of a novel care model for the management of type 2 diabetes at 1 year: an open-label, non-randomized, controlled study," *Diabetes Ther.*, vol. 9, no. 2, pp. 583–612, Apr. 2018, doi: 10.1007/s13300-018-0373-9.
14. J. Powles and H. Hodson, "Google DeepMind and healthcare in an age of algorithms," *Health Technol. (Berl).*, vol. 7, no. 4, pp. 351–367, Dec. 2017, doi: 10.1007/s12553-017-0179-1.
15. R. Vought, V. Vought, M. Shah, B. Szirth, and N. Bhagat, "EyeArt artificial intelligence analysis of diabetic retinopathy in retinal screening events," *Int. Ophthalmol.*, vol. 43, no. 12, pp. 4851–4859, Oct. 2023, doi: 10.1007/s10792-023-02887-9.
16. P. S. Rathore, A. Kumar, A. Nandal, A. Dhaka, and A. K. Sharma, "A feature explainability-based deep learning technique for diabetic foot ulcer identification," *Sci. Rep.*, vol. 15, no. 1, p. 6758, Feb. 2025, doi: 10.1038/s41598-025-90780-z.
17. P. N. Thotad, G. R. Bharamagoudar, and B. S. Anami, "Diabetic foot ulcer detection using deep learning approaches," *Sensors Int.*, vol. 4, p. 100210, 2023, doi: 10.1016/j.sintl.2022.100210.

18. P. Xie *et al.*, "An explainable machine learning model for predicting in-hospital amputation rate of patients with diabetic foot ulcer," *Int. Wound J.*, vol. 19, no. 4, pp. 910–918, May 2022, doi: 10.1111/iwj.13691.
19. M. H. Yap *et al.*, "A new mobile application for standardizing diabetic foot images," *J. Diabetes Sci. Technol.*, vol. 12, no. 1, pp. 169–173, Jan. 2018, doi: 10.1177/1932296817713761.
20. C. A. Abbott *et al.*, "Innovative intelligent insole system reduces diabetic foot ulcer recurrence at plantar sites: a prospective, randomised, proof-of-concept study," *Lancet Digit. Heal.*, vol. 1, no. 6, pp. e308–e318, Oct. 2019, doi: 10.1016/S2589-7500(19)30128-1.
21. S. Medanki *et al.*, "Artificial intelligence powered glucose monitoring and controlling system: pumping module," *World J. Exp. Med.*, vol. 14, no. 1, Mar. 2024, doi: 10.5493/wjem.v14.i1.87916.
22. B. Sheng *et al.*, "Artificial intelligence for diabetes care: current and future prospects," *Lancet Diabetes Endocrinol.*, vol. 12, no. 8, pp. 569–595, Aug. 2024, doi: 10.1016/S2213-8587(24)00154-2.
23. V. Mayya, R. N. V. P. S. Kandala, V. Gurupur, C. King, G. T. Vu, and T. T. H. Wan, "Need for an artificial intelligence-based diabetes care management system in India and the United States," *Heal. Serv. Res. Manag. Epidemiol.*, vol. 11, Jan. 2024, doi: 10.1177/23333928241275292.
24. R. Agarwal *et al.*, "Addressing algorithmic bias and the perpetuation of health inequities: an AI bias aware framework," *Heal. Policy Technol.*, vol. 12, no. 1, p. 100702, Mar. 2023, doi: 10.1016/j.hlpt.2022.100702.
25. J. Bajwa, U. Munir, A. Nori, and B. Williams, "Artificial intelligence in healthcare: transforming the practice of medicine," *Futur. Healthc. J.*, vol. 8, no. 2, pp. e188–e194, Jul. 2021, doi: 10.7861/fhj.2021-0095.
26. K. Palaniappan, E. Y. T. Lin, and S. Vogel, "Global regulatory frameworks for the use of artificial intelligence (AI) in the healthcare services sector," *Healthcare*, vol. 12, no. 5, p. 562, Feb. 2024, doi: 10.3390/healthcare12050562.
27. V. Hassija *et al.*, "Interpreting black-box models: a review on explainable artificial intelligence," *Cognit. Comput.*, vol. 16, no. 1, pp. 45–74, Jan. 2024, doi: 10.1007/s12559-023-10179-8.

# Chapter 5

# Artificial intelligence in gynecology

*Shalinee Singh, Santosh Kumar, Sundararajan V. Madihally, and Imran Khan*

## 5.1 INTRODUCTION

Artificial intelligence (AI) is a computer-based digital system that imitates the processing capabilities of human brains. This intelligent system is structured analogously to the human brain, where interconnected neural nodes known as neural networks function similarly to neurons [1]. The tremendous growth of AI in recent years has resulted in a profusion of advances in artificial neural networks (ANNs), which allow analyzing multiple data more easily using a mathematical framework. Best results are produced by these networks as the neurons are connected by multiple synapses, which facilitate the flow of data between the neurons. Assembling these various connections allows computer algorithms to replicate cognitive tasks such as problem-solving, reasoning, and so on. Various advantages of AI have led to its widespread application in the medical industry for evaluating massive data. This helps to monitor diagnosis, patients, prognosis, and prevention. In the span of the last 20 years, there has been a sharp increase in AI adoption in healthcare systems. The statistics records have shown that AI investments in medical care systems are expected to increase 18 times by 2025. However, applications of AI are interdisciplinary. Hence, for AI to be implemented successfully in healthcare systems, it is essential to collaborate in addition to basic training. AI implementations in medical service include computer-aided fetal evaluations (CAFEs), cardiotocography (CTG), and so on. The system based on individually randomized controlled trial of 46,000 women with a subset of 7,000 survived babies was intended to detect episodic variations in heart rate and fetal movements [2]. In contrast, ANNs have allowed for preliminary identification of ovarian cancer. And there have been various experiments that have been performed to predict preterm labor by studying electrohysterography (uterine electrical impulses) [2].

Amidst all of this, AI integration into in vitro fertilization (IVF) decision-making has emerged as a fertile procedure in medical centers recently. AI provides practitioners and physicians with highly reliable decision-making.

DOI: 10.1201/9781003741770-5

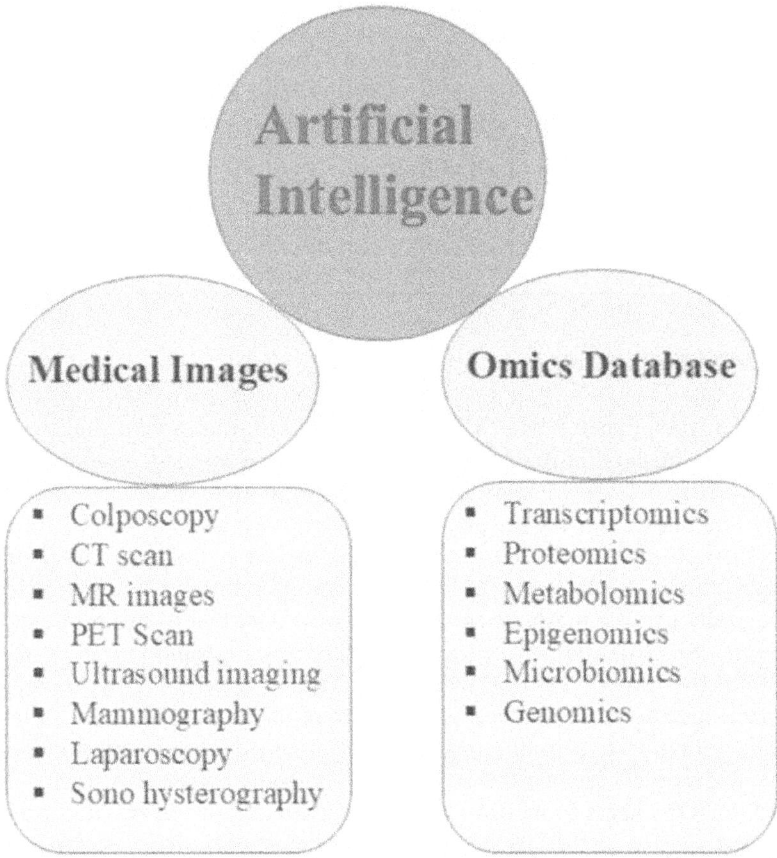


*Figure 5.1* Implementation of AI in different areas of gynecology

It is also critical to understand that AI is not a viable substitute for therapeutic applications. Overall, the reason for rampant proliferation of AI in clinical diagnosis is mortality caused by erroneous prediction and diagnosis [3]. For example, various quantitative data such as size, shape, intensity, and texture are extracted from medical images, which is referred to as radiomics (Figure 5.1). This procedure starts with image acquisition and reconstruction, then moves on to feature extraction and segmentation. The final data is assembled into an extensive database that combines histology data, serum indicators, genetic profiles, and clinical records for improved analysis [4]. This radiomics has a pivotal role in the detection of female malignancies by creating a signature profile. Hence, AI decreases errors by improving forecasting accuracy. This book chapter reviews at recent studies, advantages, drawbacks, and possible uses in gynecology [5].

## 5.2 BRIEF HISTORY OF AI

Even though there has been no specific definition of AI, its widespread use is like "information processing by a computer as human" and is defined from various perspectives based on timing and researchers. The 1950s saw the introduction of "inference and search" approaches, which led to the first wave of AI research. The formalization of AI as a separate field and the introduction of fundamental methods for problem-solving and logical reasoning defined this era, which is frequently seen as the first significant boom in AI. The phrase "artificial intelligence" was first used in this era, indicating the rise of a field devoted to the creation of computational search algorithms and machine-based thinking. The second AI boom started in the 1980s and 1990s as personal computers proliferated with the emergence of the "expert system." An expert system is a computer program designed to mimic the decision-making ability and specialized knowledge of a human expert and uses that information to solve the problem on the expert's behalf. Initially, AI researchers were hopeful that AI would eventually supplant human intelligence. However, serious limits were quickly exposed due to the difficulties in handling exceptions, resolving conflicting rules, and encoding expert knowledge into algorithms.

The discrepancy in that AI could be used everywhere, and the later discovery that AI systems needed specific instructions to work presented major obstacles to the next phase of AI development. This criticism is mostly focused on two problems: (1) AI could only solve fundamental and logic-based problem, making it useless for complex real-world applications; and (2) even when AI algorithms were used to solve real-world problems, their computational demands exceeded the processing power of the hardware at hand. Two major factors led to the emergence of the third and current AI boom after this period of disillusionment: The advancement of sophisticated machine learning methods, such as deep learning, and significant increases in processing power. It was made possible to complete hard activities, such as complex calculations and processing massive datasets, in much shorter amounts of time, especially because of the computational speedup provided by graphics processing units [6].

## 5.3 DOMAIN OF AI

### 5.3.1 Machine learning and deep learning algorithm

Both machine learning (ML) and deep learning (DL) are part of AI (Figure 5.2). ML encompasses a wide range of analytical methodologies employed in technology to identify a recurring trend and acquire predictive criteria from data and categorize unknown objects [7].

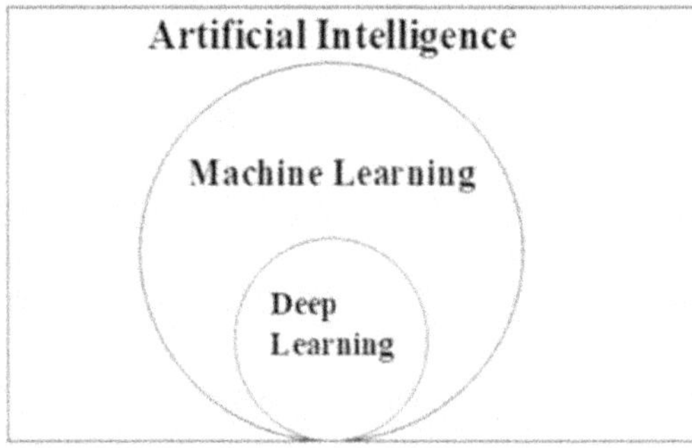


*Figure 5.2* Connections among AI, DL, and ML. An outline of how DL and ML are integrated with AI. While DL is a subset of AI that uses mathematical and statistical models, AI itself is an area that mimics human intelligence through machines and algorithms

DL is a subset of ML and a major force behind the current developments in AI. DL is based on ANN computational models modeled after the composition and operations of organic neurons in the human brain. Similar to the nervous system, several layers of filters provide an output that serves as input to the next layers. Input layers, hidden (or intermediate) layers, and output layers are the three main layers that make up an ANN. Each of these layer categories may contain more than one layer. The output of the network is compared to the anticipated outcomes obtained from the training data during the learning phase. For the reduction of inaccuracy and improvement of the precision of subsequent predictions, the model modifies the weights assigned to the connections between neurons based on this comparison. The introduction of DL has enabled the potential to use in image recognition, anomaly detection, and language processing [6, 8]. Some have utilized DL for automating placental segmentation on imaging during gestational age [9]. In particular, convolutional neural networks (CNNs) have been adapted extensively in reproductive medicine due to the possibility of determining the probability of success in the in vitro fertilization. These are built using data from various steps such as image analysis of sperm injection puncture position and embryonic chromosomal data estimation [10–12].

Transfer learning is a DL approach that enhances learning efficiency by applying results obtained from one domain to another or a previously unseen domain.

Supervised learning, unsupervised learning, and reinforcement learning are three major types of ML (Figure 5.3). The development of prediction models using labeled training data is known as supervised learning, and it is mostly used for tasks like classification and regression analysis. This paradigm makes it easier to build a model that can produce suitable outputs

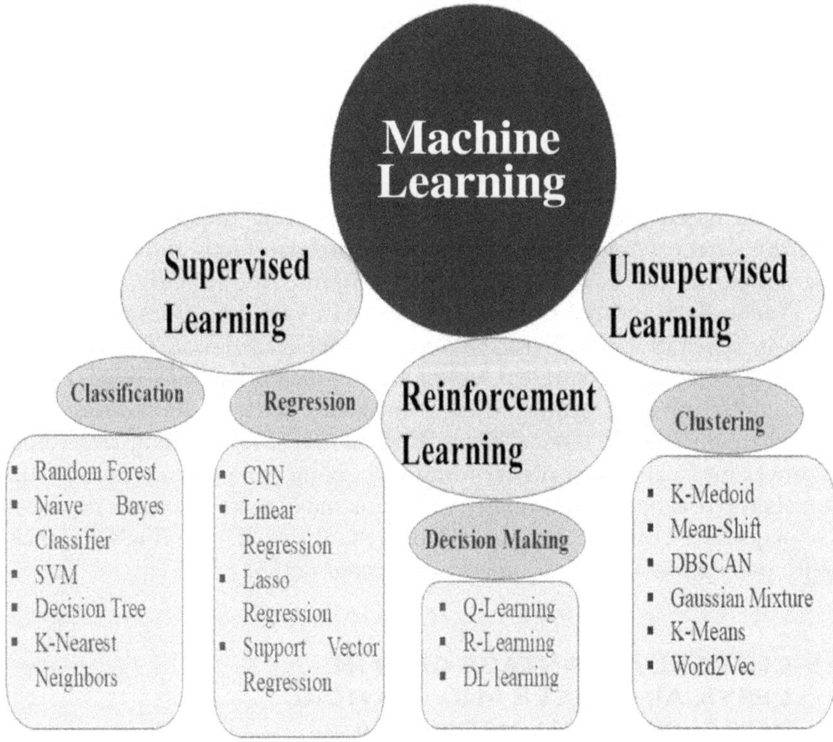


*Figure 5.3* Classification of machine learning algorithms

for novel, unseen inputs by using the training data as reference information. Regression analysis in its different forms and decision tree-based algorithms, such as the random forest algorithm, is a prominent method in supervised learning. Random forest algorithm consists of many decision trees mimicking a forest, and it is used for regression analysis as well as classification. Supervised learning makes up more than 90% of DL applications.

Contrary to supervised learning, unsupervised learning does not rely on predetermined outputs to direct the learning process and does not employ labeled training data. Rather, it looks for underlying patterns, structures, or groupings in the data to provide insights on how it is organized [6, 8]. Clustering is one of the most used techniques in unsupervised learning.

Reinforcement learning develops algorithms that find better choices and actions through trial and error [6]. One could state that reinforcement learning may be a combination of supervised and unsupervised learning. Reinforcement learning algorithms learn how to complete tasks using a set of decisions that are not explicitly instructed.

## 5.4 CLINICAL ADVANTAGE OF AI IN GYNECOLOGY

The adoption of AI in gynecology has grown in popularity, especially in the interpretation of fetal heart rate monitoring and cardiotocography (CTG). AI helps with preterm labor prediction, pregnancy problem identification, and physician clinical interpretation discrepancies. These developments help to lower the morbidity and mortality rates among mothers and newborns. AI has a great deal of promise for creating predictive algorithms that can detect women who are at risk of preterm birth and not showing any symptoms and have shorter cervical lengths. Additionally, by combining genetic data and multiomics analysis, AI's vast data storage capacities make it easier to identify risk factors for premature labor. Consequently, this helps to optimize surgical techniques, reduce pregnancy-related problems, and improve surgeon training in authentic settings. By creating materials that mimic real tissues, three-dimensional (3D) printing technology improves medical education even more by giving students access to lifelike models for practice. Additionally, surgeons may create accurate preoperative plans based on tissue size and depth, thanks to 3D imaging's enhanced depth perception over two-dimensional imaging [13].

## 5.5 CLINICAL ADVANTAGE OF AI IN CERVICAL CANCER AND CERVICAL INTRAEPITHELIAL NEOPLASIA

AI has been used in numerous research studies on cervical cancer and cervical intraepithelial neoplasia (CIN). These studies can be mainly categorized into the analysis of data from cytology, magnetic resonance imaging (MRI), CT, colposcopy, and human papillomavirus (HPV) [14].

### 5.5.1 Pap smear and HPV testing

Cervical cancer holds the fourth rank in most prevalent malignancy among women on the global scale, with an estimated 569,847 newly reported cases and 311,365 associated deaths annually [15]. A report issued by the World Health Organization (WHO) estimates that 350,000 women worldwide lost their lives to cervical cancer in 2022, while 660,000 women received a diagnosis. The remarkable differences in access to treatment and preventive measures are highlighted by the fact that more than 94% of these deaths are in economically emerging countries [16]. The expected death toll from cervical cancer in India increased gradually from 32,246 in 2019 to 35,691 in 2023. These figures demonstrate how urgently improved screening, immunization, and treatment initiatives are needed to alleviate the worldwide cervical cancer burden. However, it is the second most frequent malignancy in Indian women, with a rate of 14.7–24.3 per 100,000. As liquid-based cytology facilities are limited, most screening centers continue to use Papanicolaou-stained traditional smears. Manual screening is time-consuming, and automated solutions could boost efficiency by detecting problems for pathologist assessment. While such devices exist for liquid cytology, none are available for traditional smears [17]. Several deep learning experiments incorporating pathological pictures of cervical cancer or CIN use cytology (Pap smears). In another study, a model was developed that identified normal and abnormal results in 1,838 cervical cytology photos using deep learning (normal 1,301 and abnormal 537 images). The results indicated 94% accuracy, 96% sensitivity, and 91% specificity. Another study analyzed 700,000 cytologic pictures using deep learning and created a model to recognize tumors with a CIN $\geq 2$. The AI-assisted diagnostic accuracy was greater in comparison to the unassisted one [17]. AI research has also classified the severity of CIN and cancer in situ [6]. Another AI-assisted cytology system was assessed in a prospective cohort study that involved 0.7 million women in a cervical cancer screening program: 94.7% (with 0.92 kappa value) of the 98,549 instances that were screened using both AI and manual approaches agreed. In Atypical Squamous Cells-High grade lesion (Odds Ratio = 1.22, $p < 0.001$) and High-grade Squamous Intraepithelial Lesion (HSIL) (Odds Ratio = 1.41, $p < 0.001$) cases, AI showed increased detection rates for CIN2+, with 5.8% higher sensitivity than manual reading, albeit with a little decrease in specificity. These results support the use of AI-based cytology to screen for cervical cancer on a broad scale, improving sensitivity while preserving clinical dependability [18].

These AI-assisted diagnosis methodologies increased specificity, maintaining sensitivity in human papilloma virus-positive patients. Tian et al. [15] developed a 39 Mb capture panel that was created specifically to target 522 genes commonly altered in cervical cancer and 17 strains of the human papillomavirus (HPV). In order to evaluate the HPV integration status, somatic mutations, and copy number variations (CNVs), this panel was used in a capture-based next-generation sequencing analysis of 34 matched clinical samples. Ten HPV-positive (HPV+) cases, 10 instances with CIN of various grades, and 14 cases with CIN2+ [including CIN2 ($n = 1$), CIN2–3 ($n = 3$), CIN3 ($n = 9$), and squamous cell carcinoma ($n = 1$)] were included in the sample cohort. Biomarkers enriched in CIN2+ were incorporated into a risk classification model for cervical precursor lesions using the Recency, Frequency and Monetary (RFM) learning technique. Non-synonymous somatic mutations (2 in CIN1, 12 in CIN2+), CNVs (19.1 in HPV+, 29.4 in CIN1, and 127 in CIN2+), and HPV integration events (11 in HPV+, 25 in CIN1, and 56 in CIN2+) all gradually increased, according to the data, suggesting a relationship with the advancement of the disease. The mitochondrial chromosome was considerably and frequently lost in CIN2+ instances

($p = 0.009$), which may indicate that it plays a part in cervical neoplastic transformation. CIN2+ individuals had a large "common" loss of the mitochondrial chromosome ($p = 0.009$). CIN2+ enhanced biomarkers, including HPV information, mutation, amplification, mitochondrial alteration, and deletion, accurately predicted CIN2+ with an accuracy of 0.814 [15].

### 5.5.2 AI in colposcopy

In a study, Sato et al. implemented deep learning to 485 colposcopy pictures to indicate strong possibilities of CIN. The validation set had a diagnosis accuracy of approximately 50%. Another study employed colposcopy photos from a cohort of 19,435 patients across multiple centers to create a deep learning model for colposcopy-based diagnosis and a biopsy guidance system called the colposcopic AI auxiliary diagnostic system. Biopsy evaluations by this approach were substantially more accurate than those performed by gynecologists (82.2% vs. 65.9%; area under the curve (AUC) 0.750 vs. 0.516; $p < 0.001$). Since there are only a few photographs available, attempts are made to improve accuracy. Transfer learning is a DL technique that enhances learning efficiency by applying knowledge gained from one domain to a different, previously unseen domain [19]. Kudva et al. [20] devised a hybrid transfer learning method, which has improved the accuracy to 91% for colposcopy picture identification using their deep learning system. Other cervical imaging methods geared at AI-based diagnosis system have been developed [20]. Hu et al. [21] created cervicography, a method in which a camera targets cervical lesions and utilizes deep learning to interpret the images. With a 91% accuracy rate, the data indicate that cervicography may become a viable method for screening of cervical cancer. Some deep learning algorithms have also integrated HPV testing data to improve diagnostic performance, going beyond AI applications that only use colposcopic pictures [21].

### 5.5.3 AI in MRI and CT scan

A common technique for assessing localized cervical cancer is magnetic resonance imaging (MRI). New research has investigated using AI to improve diagnostic precision. A DL-based model was used to analyze sagittal and T2-weighted MRI scans of the uterus from 241 control people and 177 patients with cervical cancer in a study by Urushibara et al. The findings demonstrated the AI model's potential as a helpful aid in clinical decision-making by showing that its diagnostic performance was on par with that of qualified radiologists [22]. In another study, Liu et al. [23] examined 1,193 cervical cancer patients treated with intensity-modulated radiotherapy (IMRT) from 2011 to 2015, separating them into two cohorts: development (797) and validation (396). The two-year distant metastasis rates

(DMR) were 12.8% and 13.3%, respectively. Non-squamous cell cancer, common iliac LNM, and bilateral pelvic LNM were revealed as significant risk factors. Patients with two to three risk factors showed significantly greater DMR (39.3% vs. 19.3%, $p < 0.001$; 47.6% vs. 10.9%, $p < 0.001$). A predictive algorithm was created to detect high-risk individuals and provide improved clinical care. Wu et al. [24] created another method using preoperative MRI data from a total of 894 patients with stage IB and IIB cervical cancer going through radical hysterectomy, a DL model that was created to forecast lymph node metastases. The model had a 75% accuracy rate, 88% sensitivity, and 71% specificity after being trained on tumor lesions and circumferential characteristics in T1-weighted images. In addition, there has been research into using AI to analyze computed tomography (CT) pictures of cervical cancer. Using CT imaging features and chemosensitivity data from 221 patients, a random forest algorithm was used to create a predictive chemoresponse modeling framework in locally advanced cervical cancer. This method showed strong predictive performance with an AUC value of 0.821, demonstrating the promise of AI in maximizing treatment plans for cervical cancer [24].

## 5.6 CLINICAL ADVANTAGE OF AI IN ENDOMETRIAL CANCER

The rising incidence and death from endometrial cancer are cause for concern, particularly in fast-transitioning societies with the highest rates. The Federation of Gynecology and Obstetrics or popularly referred to as (FIGO) staging system is used for surgical and pathological classification. The majority of endometrial cancer patients (80% at stage I) are detected early, with five-year patient survival statistics of more than 95%, the highest among gynecological cancers [25]. Only a few research studies have employed AI in endometrial cancer in comparison to ovarian and cervical cancer. These research studies are classified into two categories: clinical database reports and medical imaging reports among patients of endometrial cancer [6].

### 5.6.1 Medical imaging

MRI is a critical part of the pre-surgical evaluation of endometrial cancer, and deep learning algorithms are being investigated for application. Deep muscle invasion serves as a crucial indicator of prognosis in uterine cancer. Dong et al. [26] used 4,896 MR images from 72 endometrial cancer patients from multiple centers to train a DL model that predicted deep muscle invasion and compared its performance to radiologist's evaluations. Both approaches have accuracy rates of 75% or greater, with no statistically significant difference between them [26]. A retrospective analysis examined MRI data (2015–2020) of endometrial cancer or non-cancerous lesion patients. In Experiment 1, a convolutional neural network (CNN) was trained on individual and combined image datasets from 204 cancer and 184 non-cancerous cases, then tested on 97 images (51 cancer, 46 non-cancerous), with interpretations provided by three blinded radiologists. Experiment 2 examined whether adding different image kinds enhanced CNN diagnostic performance. The AUC values for CNNs employing individual and combined picture sets ranged 0.88–0.95 and 0.87–0.93, respectively, demonstrating comparable performance to radiologists. The use of several image kinds resulted in an AUC of 0.88–0.95, validating CNN effectiveness [27]. In other work, Chen et al. [28] collected 530 MRI scans from 4,806 endometrial cancer patients to create a DL model for predicting deep muscle invasion. Findings of the study revealed 84% precision, 66.7% sensitivity, and 87.5% specificity. As lymph node metastasis helps determine treatment strategy and patient outcome, pre-surgical evaluation through imaging for endometrial cancer is critical [28].

### 5.6.2 Clinical information (databases)

DL methods have been applied to endometrial cancer datasets in a number of studies. One such study evaluated the viability of classifying patients into four molecular subtypes using a random forest algorithm in conjunction with data from 13 next-generation sequencing gene panels and microsatellite instability (MSI) tests. The diagnostic accuracy of the model was 0.9753. According to these findings, clinical genetic panel testing may make it easier to categorize patients into four different prognostic groups. For the examination, a total of 96 formalin-fixed paraffin-embedded samples were sequenced using the next-generation sequencing TruSeq Custom Amplicon low-input procedure (Illumina) along with a multi-gene panel. MSI analysis was carried out through fragment analysis with eight microsatellite markers. The random forest algorithm successfully classified endometrial cancer patients using next-generation sequencing data into TCGA prognostic subtypes with 97.53% accuracy ($p < 0.001$) for CNH and CNL classification. The prognostic relevance of these groups was validated for disease-free survival of $p = 0.004$ and overall survival of $p = 0.030$, establishing this method as an accurate tool for endometrial cancer prediction [29].

In another study, ML was used to create predictive models for lymph node metastases using pathology data from 762 endometrial cancer patients by Günakan et al. [30]. Vascular invasion, tissue type, tumor diameter, myometrial invasion depth, cervical involvement, and adnexal metastasis were among the variables. For lymph node metastases, the final model showed a prediction accuracy of almost 85%. A different study examined the differences between classification and regression trees (CARTs) and ANNs in the detection of endometrial cancer. Among the 178 participants in the study were 72 healthy postmenopausal controls and 106 women with endometrial cancer diagnoses. The clinical factors analyzed included age, menopause status, diabetes, hypertension, smoking, and obesity. ANNs outperformed CARTs, which had a diagnostic accuracy of 77.5%, with an accuracy of 85.4%. These results highlight the promise of ANN-based methods for better endometrial cancer diagnosis [31].

## 5.7 CLINICAL ADVANTAGE OF AI IN OVARIAN CANCER

Ovarian cancer, which has a high death rate among gynecological cancers, is difficult to detect early because of its frequently mild symptoms and the dearth of reliable screening techniques. With an aim of enhancing outcomes for patients, AI holds promise in the analysis of complex medical data, including imaging, genetic information, and clinical records.

### 5.7.1 Medical images

MRI is a critical part of the pre-surgical evaluation of malignant and benign ovarian tumors. Wang et al. [32] implemented a new algorithm for identifying benign or malignant tumors by evaluating MR images of 451 ovarian tumor patients using deep learning and contrasting the program's output with radiologists' interpretations. Higher accuracy (0.87 vs. 0.64, with $p < 0.001$), specificity (0.92 vs. 0.64, with $p < 0.001$), and comparable sensitivity (0.75 vs. 0.63, with $p = 0.407$) were shown by the established diagnosis model that combined MR images with clinical data. Another helpful method for differentiating between non-malignant and malignant ovarian tumors is ultrasound, and deep learning has been used in numerous research [32]. In another study, DL research made use of CT scans. Wang et al. created a pattern predicting framework by evaluating 8,917 CT scans collected from 245 malignant serous carcinomas cases. The two cohort studies, with accuracy values of 0.722 and 0.694, were utilized for the determination of accuracy and recurrence prediction at three years. Various other studies have also utilized CT images for DL [33].

### 5.7.2 Database of clinical information

There have been various studies on ovarian cancer that have been examined through ML algorithms employing clinical information data. In the treatment of ovarian cancer, it is critical to evaluate the anticipated effectiveness of R0 resection prior to its implementation. In a study, Laios et al. [34] created a prediction model for the R0 surgery success rate using the k-nearest neighbors classifier and clinical data as parameters such as age, BMI, CA 125, clinical difficulty score, Charlson comorbidity index, disease score, and operative procedure. The findings revealed a negative predictive value of over 90% and an accuracy rate of 66% [34]. In another study, Akazawa et al. used a predictive model for differentiating between non-malignant and malignant ovarian cancers that was created using five machine learning algorithms with clinical and computed tomography (CT) scan data. Age, menopause status, endometriosis, BMI, hemoglobin levels, leukocyte count, C-reactive protein, CA 125, and CA 19-9 were among the clinical factors. Tumor size and the presence or absence of ascites were included in the CT scan data. Data from 202 ovarian tumor patients, 23 with indeterminate malignancy, 53 with cancer, and 126 with benign tumors were used to train the model. Among the five ways, the machine learning algorithm known as XG-Boost had the greatest correct diagnosis rate (0.80) [35].

### 5.7.3 Databases of omics

Applications of AI to basic research datasets, like omics analysis, have also been made in ovarian cancer research. The identification of neoplastic cells and cytotoxic T lymphocytes is necessary for immunotherapy to be effective. Nevertheless, little is known about the variables affecting the T cells' geographic distribution inside the microenvironment of the tumor.

Desbois and coworkers [36] analyzed a large cohort of ovarian cancer data using transcriptome data and pathological pictures, developing a machine learning approach to molecularly categorize and define tumor immunophenotypes. In a study, Matsuo et al. [37] examined comprehensive blood glycopeptide spectra analysis (CSGSA), a method that uses supervised modeling to find distinctive patterns in over 10,000 blood glycopeptides. The findings show the higher accuracy of CSGSA than CA125 and HE4 in diagnosing initial-stage epithelial ovarian cancer. And the combination of CSGSA, CA125, and HE4 had enhanced the diagnostic efficacy, pointing to CSGSA as a viable screening method for the preliminary diagnosis of ovarian cancer. Tanabe et al. [38] processed data from AI-driven comprehensive serum glycopeptide spectra analysis (CSGSA-AI) approach that used a CNN to identify irregular glycans in epithelial ovarian cancer (EOC) patients. Serum glycopeptide profiling was transformed into 2D barcodes, allowing for CNN-based classification of EOC and non-EOC samples. The model was trained on 60% of the samples and verified on 40%, and glycopeptide alignment using principal component analysis increased diagnostic accuracy to 88%. When the CNN was trained using 2D barcodes color-coded by CA125 and HE4 serum levels, its accuracy climbed to 95%. This low-cost, high-accuracy technique has the potential to improve EOC detection [38].

### 5.7.4 AI in reproductive technology, polycystic ovary syndrome

Different models had been created to automatically partition or measure ovarian follicles, assess ovarian volume, and track follicular growth over time in the majority of studies (6 out of 11) involving infertile women receiving assisted reproductive technology (ART) [39]. Using 2D or 3D ultrasound pictures as the model parameter, these experiments created either DL models ($n$ = 5) [40] or ML models ($n$ = 1), and they demonstrated good-to-high DICE performance. Both ultrasonography and clinical data were used as model inputs in two studies that created models to predict hyper-responsiveness during ART cycles. In a study, the ML model had an AUC of 0.91, while the DL model had an AUC of 0.88 in the other study. An accuracy of 0.94 was reported by one study that used amplitude- and frequency-based features to create an ML model that could distinguish between a favorable and unfavorable uterine cavity for embryo implantation. In a study by Li et al. [41], the AUC of 0.89 was shown in one study that created a machine learning model to assess endometrial elasticity as determined by shear-wave elastography in infertility patients that cannot be explained. In another study, Bones et al. [42] collected the 3D ultrasound scans from women with a history of repeated spontaneous miscarriage, infertile women, and women in the general population, who experienced repeated spontaneous miscarriages. After that, a DL model was created for segmentation and alignment of uterine shape, and it performed well in terms of DICE (0.90). In order to differentiate between normal ovaries/ovarian cysts and PCOS on ultrasonography, a few studies created ML models ($n$ = 7), DL models ($n$ = 3), or both ($n$ = 2) [43]. Shape, intensity, clinical, geometrical, ultrasonic, morphological, stereological, statistical, and textural feature families were among the feature families that were used as model inputs in the models. Eleven studies reported the model's performance as an accuracy score (varying from 0.82 to 0.99), whereas one study reported it as an F1 score (0.76) [42, 44].

## 5.8 CONCLUSION

AI research in gynecologic malignancies has grown significantly over the last few years with applications in genomic and clinical data processing, as well as medical imaging (CT, MRI, and cytopathology). However, a few AI-driven findings have been successfully applied in clinical practice despite encouraging developments, underscoring the need for additional study and validation to strengthen AI's position in gynecology. AI has also been incorporated into gynecological screening processes to reduce the possibility of undetected lesions. AI's capacity to lessen radiologists' workload by improving computer image processing for effective lesion diagnosis is one of its main benefits. To provide individualized follow-up care and screening methods, mammography computer vision technology may eventually be implemented into decision support systems to customize follow-up care and screening methods for each patient.

## ACKNOWLEDGMENTS

This chapter was supported by Harcourt Butler Technical University in 2024.

## LIST OF ABBREVIATIONS

| | |
|---|---|
| ANN | artificial neural network |
| ART | assisted reproductive technology |
| AUC | area under the curve |
| BMI | body mass index |
| CA | cancer antigen |
| CAFE | computer-aided fetal evaluation |
| CART | classification and regression tree |
| CIN | cervical intraepithelial neoplasia |
| CNH | copy number high |
| CNL | copy number low |
| CNN | convolutional neural network |
| CTG | cardiotocography |
| CSGSA | comprehensive serum glycopeptide spectra analysis |
| CT | computed tomography |
| DICE | differentiable image computing engine |
| DL | deep learning |
| DMR | distant metastasis rate |
| EOC | epithelial ovarian cancer |
| HE4 | human epididymis protein 4 |
| HPV | human papillomavirus |
| IVF | in vitro fertilization |
| LNM | lymph node metastasis |
| ML | machine learning |
| MRI | magnetic resonance imaging |
| MSI | microsatellite instability |
| PCOS | polycystic ovary syndrome |
| TCGA | The Cancer Genome Atlas |
| XG-Boost | extreme gradient boosting |

## REFERENCES

1. P. Iftikhar, M. Kuijpers, A. Khayyat, and M. Sa, "Artificial intelligence: a new paradigm in obstetrics and gynecology research and clinical practice," *Cureus*, Feb. 2020, https://doi.org/10.7759/cureus.7124.
2. P. Brocklehurst and on behalf of T. I. C. Group, "A study of an intelligent system to support decision making in the management of labour using the cardiotocograph – the INFANT study protocol," *BMC Pregnancy Childbirth*, vol. 16, no. 1, p. 10, 2016, https://doi.org/10.1186/s12884-015-0780-0.
3. M. A. Makary and M. Daniel, "Medical error—the third leading cause of death in the US," *BMJ*, vol. 353, p. i2139, May 2016, https://doi.org/10.1136/bmj.i2139.
4. M. A. Wahed, M. Alqaraleh, M. S. Alzboon, and M. S. Al Batah, "Application of artificial intelligence for diagnosing tumors in the female reproductive system: a systematic review," *Multidisciplinar (Montevideo)*, vol. 54, no. 3, p. 15, 2025.
5. P. Shrestha *et al.*, "A systematic review on the use of artificial intelligence in gynecologic imaging – Background, state of the art, and future directions," *Gynecol Oncol*, vol. 166, no. 3, pp. 596–605, Sep. 2022, https://doi.org/10.1016/j.ygyno.2022.07.024.
6. K. Sone *et al.*, "Application of artificial intelligence in gynecologic malignancies: A review," *J Obstet Gynaecol Res*, vol. 47, no. 8, pp. 2577–2585, Aug. 2021, https://doi.org/10.1111/jog.14818.
7. S. A. Shazly, E. C. Trabuco, C. G. Ngufor, and A. O. Famuyide, "Introduction to machine learning in obstetrics and gynecology," *Obstet Gynecol*, vol. 139, no. 4, pp. 669–679, 2022.
8. F. Emmert-Streib, Z. Yang, H. Feng, S. Tripathi, and M. Dehmer, "An introductory review of deep learning for prediction models with big data," *Front Artif Intell*, vol. 3, 2020, [Online]. Available: https://www.frontiersin.org/journals/artificial-intelligence/articles/10.3389/frai.2020.00004
9. Z. Liu Y and Y. R. F, "Evaluation of spatial attentive deep learning for automatic placental segmentation on longitudinal MRI," *J Magn Reson Imaging*, vol. 57, no. 5, pp. 1533–1540, 2023.
10. C. L. Curchoe, A. Flores-Saiffe Farias, G. Mendizabal-Ruiz, and A. Chavez-Badiola, "Evaluating predictive models in reproductive medicine," *Fertil Steril*, vol. 114, no. 5, pp. 921–926, 2020, https://doi.org/10.1016/j.fertnstert.2020.09.159.
11. M. Zhou *et al.*, "Apoptotic bodies for advanced drug delivery and therapy," *Journal of Controlled Release*, vol. 351, pp. 394–406, 2022, https://doi.org/10.1016/j.jconrel.2022.09.045.
12. K. Kitaya *et al.*, "Construction of deep learning-based convolutional neural network model for automatic detection of fluid hysteroscopic endometrial micropolyps in infertile women with chronic endometritis," *Eur J Obstet Gynecol Reprod Biol*, vol. 297, pp. 249–253, 2024, https://doi.org/10.1016/j.ejogrb.2024.04.026.
13. S. N. Malani IV, D. Shrivastava, and M. S. Raka, "A comprehensive review of the role of artificial intelligence in obstetrics and gynecology," *Cureus*, vol. 15, no. 2, 2023.
14. N. Bizzarri *et al.*, "Radiomics systematic review in cervical cancer: gynecological oncologists' perspective," *Int J Gynecol Cancer*, vol. 33, no. 10, pp. 1522–1541, 2023, https://doi.org/10.1136/ijgc-2023-004589.

15. R. Tian *et al.*, "Risk stratification of cervical lesions using capture sequencing and machine learning method based on HPV and human integrated genomic profiles," *Carcinogenesis*, vol. 40, no. 10, pp. 1220–1228, Oct. 2019, https://doi.org/10.1093/carcin/bgz094.
16. World Health Organization, *Cervical cancer fact sheet*, World Health Organization, Mar. 2024.
17. P. Sanyal, P. Ganguli, and S. Barui, "Performance characteristics of an artificial intelligence based on convolutional neural network for screening conventional Papanicolaou-stained cervical smears," *Med J Armed Forces India*, vol. 76, no. 4, pp. 418–424, 2020, https://doi.org/10.1016/j.mjafi.2019.08.001.
18. H. Bao *et al.*, "The artificial intelligence-assisted cytology diagnostic system in large-scale cervical cancer screening: A population-based cohort study of 0.7 million women," *Cancer Med*, vol. 9, no. 18, pp. 6896–6906, Sep. 2020, https://doi.org/10.1002/cam4.3296.
19. M. Sato *et al.*, "Application of deep learning to the classification of images from colposcopy," *Oncol Lett*, vol. 15, Jan. 2018, https://doi.org/10.3892/ol.2018.7762.
20. V. Kudva, K. Prasad, and S. Guruvare, "Hybrid transfer learning for classification of uterine cervix images for cervical cancer screening," *J Digit Imaging*, vol. 33, pp. 619–631, 2019, [Online]. Available: https://api.semanticscholar.org/CorpusID:209392881
21. L. Hu *et al.*, "An observational study of deep learning and automated evaluation of cervical images for cancer screening," *Obstet Gynecol Surv*, 2019, [Online]. Available: https://api.semanticscholar.org/CorpusID:58616165
22. A. Urushibara *et al.*, "Diagnosing uterine cervical cancer on a single T2-weighted image: Comparison between deep learning versus radiologists.," *Eur J Radiol*, vol. 135, p. 109471, 2020, [Online]. Available: https://api.semanticscholar.org/CorpusID:229324601
23. X. Liu, Q. Meng, W. Wang, Z. Zhou, F. Zhang, and K. Hu, "Predictors of distant metastasis in patients with cervical cancer treated with definitive radiotherapy," *J Cancer*, vol. 10, no. 17, pp. 3967–3974, 2019, https://doi.org/10.7150/jca.31538.
24. Q. Wu *et al.*, "Development of a deep learning model to identify lymph node metastasis on magnetic resonance imaging in patients with cervical cancer," *JAMA Netw Open*, vol. 3, no. 7, pp. e2011625–e2011625, Jul. 2020, https://doi.org/10.1001/jamanetworkopen.2020.11625.
25. V. Bhardwaj *et al.*, "Machine learning for endometrial cancer prediction and prognostication," *Front Oncol*, vol. 12, 2022, [Online]. Available: https://www.frontiersin.org/journals/oncology/articles/10.3389/fonc.2022.852746
26. H.-C. Dong, H.-K. Dong, M.-H. Yu, Y.-H. Lin, and C.-C. Chang, "Using deep learning with convolutional neural network approach to identify the invasion depth of endometrial cancer in myometrium using MR images: a pilot study," *Int J Environ Res Public Health*, vol. 17, no. 16, 2020, https://doi.org/10.3390/ijerph17165993.
27. A. Urushibara *et al.*, "The efficacy of deep learning models in the diagnosis of endometrial cancer using MRI: a comparison with radiologists," *BMC Med Imaging*, vol. 22, no. 1, p. 80, 2022, https://doi.org/10.1186/s12880-022-00808-3.

28. X. Chen *et al.*, "Deep learning for the determination of myometrial invasion depth and automatic lesion identification in endometrial cancer MR imaging: a preliminary study in a single institution," *Eur Radiol*, vol. 30, Apr. 2020, https://doi.org/10.1007/s00330-020-06870-1.
29. R. López-Reig *et al.*, "Prognostic classification of endometrial cancer using a molecular approach based on a twelve-gene NGS panel," *Sci Rep*, vol. 9, no. 1, p. 18093, 2019, https://doi.org/10.1038/s41598-019-54624-x.
30. A. S. H. A. K. İ. G. E. A. A. Günakan E, "A novel prediction method for lymph node involvement in endometrial cancer: machine learning," *Int J Gynecol Cancer*, vol. 29, no. 2, pp. 320–324, 2019.
31. V. Pergialiotis *et al.*, "The utility of artificial neural networks and classification and regression trees for the prediction of endometrial cancer in postmenopausal women," *Public Health*, vol. 164, pp. 1–6, 2018, [Online]. Available: https://api.semanticscholar.org/CorpusID:52127068
32. R. Wang *et al.*, "Evaluation of a convolutional neural network for ovarian tumor differentiation based on magnetic resonance imaging," *Eur Radiol*, vol. 31, no. 7, pp. 4960–4971, 2021, https://doi.org/10.1007/s00330-020-07266-x.
33. S. Wang *et al.*, "Deep learning provides a new computed tomography-based prognostic biomarker for recurrence prediction in high-grade serous ovarian cancer," *Radiother Oncol J Europ Soc Therapeutic Radiother Oncol*, vol. 132, pp. 171–177, 2019.
34. A. Laios, A. Gryparis, D. DeJong, R. Hutson, G. Theophilou, and C. Leach, "Predicting complete cytoreduction for advanced ovarian cancer patients using nearest-neighbor models," *J Ovarian Res*, vol. 13, no. 1, p. 117, 2020, https://doi.org/10.1186/s13048-020-00700-0.
35. M. Akazawa and K. Hashimoto, "Artificial intelligence in gynecologic cancers: Current status and future challenges – A systematic review," *Artif Intell Med*, vol. 120, p. 102164, 2021, https://doi.org/10.1016/j.artmed.2021.102164.
36. M. Desbois *et al.*, "Integrated digital pathology and transcriptome analysis identifies molecular mediators of T-cell exclusion in ovarian cancer," *Nat Commun*, vol. 11, no. 1, p. 5583, 2020, https://doi.org/10.1038/s41467-020-19408-2.
37. K. Matsuo *et al.*, "Utility of comprehensive serum glycopeptide spectra analysis (CSGSA) for the detection of early stage epithelial ovarian cancer," *Cancers (Basel)*, vol. 12, no. 9, 2020, https://doi.org/10.3390/cancers12092374.
38. K. Tanabe *et al.*, "Comprehensive serum glycopeptide spectra analysis combined with artificial intelligence (CSGSA-AI) to diagnose early-stage ovarian cancer," *Cancers (Basel)*, vol. 12, no. 9, p. 2373, 2020.
39. F. Moro *et al.*, "Application of artificial intelligence to ultrasound imaging for benign gynecological disorders: systematic review," *Ultrasound in Obstetrics & Gynecology*, Jan. 2025, https://doi.org/10.1002/uog.29171.
40. D. Srivastava, S. Gupta, S. Kudavelly, V. S. K., and R. Ga, "Unsupervised deep learning based longitudinal follicular growth tracking during IVF Cycle using 3D transvaginal ultrasound in assisted reproduction," 2021 43rd Annual International Conference of the IEEE Engineering in Medicine & Biology Society (EMBC), 2021, pp. 3209–3212, https://doi.org/10.1109/EMBC46164.2021.9630495.

41. Z. Li *et al.*, "Evaluation of endometrial receptivity in women with unexplained infertility by shear wave elastography," *Insights Imaging*, vol. 15, no. 1, p. 85, 2024, https://doi.org/10.1186/s13244-024-01646-3.
42. E. Boneš, M. Gergolet, C. Bohak, Ž. Lesar and M. Marolt, "Automatic segmentation and alignment of uterine shapes from 3D ultrasound data.," *Comput Biol Med*, vol. 178, p. 178, 2024.
43. M. Sumathi, P. Chitra, S. Sheela, and C. Ishwarya, "Study and implementation of automated system for detection of PCOS from ultrasound scan images using artificial intelligence," *The Imaging Science Journal*, vol. 72, no. 7, pp. 828–839, Oct. 2024, https://doi.org/10.1080/13682199.2023.2229016.
44. K. V, S. S, M. M. Ramya, and K. S. Sankaran, "An intelligent machine learning approach for ovarian detection and classification system using ultrasonogram images," *Engineered Science*, vol. 23, p. 879, 2023, https://doi.org/10.30919/es8d879.

Chapter 6

# Role of AI in gastroenterology

## Prevention, diagnostics, and treatment

*Imran Khan, Brajesh Kumar Khare, Mohammad Shoaib Khan, and Santosh Kumar*

### 6.1 INTRODUCTION

As artificial intelligence (AI) advances swiftly in the field of medicine, its practical uses in clinical settings are becoming more and more apparent [1]. With a strong dependence on endoscopic and radiologic imaging, gastroenterology emerges as a promising domain for AI integration. Significant attention has been directed toward various areas within this field, such as aiding in the swift diagnosis of gastrointestinal neoplastic lesions, minimizing diagnostic errors, enhancing imaging quality, reducing variability in visual classifications among observers, and refining interpretation of radiologic and histopathologic findings [2]. AI serves as an umbrella term encompassing various disciplines like machine learning (ML) and specific techniques such as deep learning (DL). The core objective of ML revolves around leveraging extensive datasets to identify patterns of interactions among variables, typically enabling the learned function to be generalized for application to new data [3]. Within ML, there exist both "supervised" and "unsupervised" learning methods. Supervised learning aims to forecast a labeled output, primarily focusing on categorizing input data into distinct subgroups or, alternatively, predicting quantitative outcomes [4]. In supervised learning, a system is trained to help identify gastric intestinal metaplasia (GIM) by utilizing a vast database of lesions previously identified by an operator as corresponding to GIM. Conversely, unsupervised learning lacks a specific output to predict. It focuses on discerning naturally occurring patterns from the input data, often for the purpose of grouping them accordingly [4]. DL operates as a subset of ML, grounded in artificial neural network (ANN) that draws loose inspiration from the interconnections of neurons in the human brain. DL autonomously learns, identifies, and harnesses predictive factors of an outcome from the input data. This process often involves the use of multi-layered systems, such as convolutional neural network (CNN), to effectively process intricate information [5]. Recent advancements in specialized computer hardware, such as enhanced graphics processing unit capabilities, alongside software and algorithmic breakthroughs, have made the realization of DL feasible. The

DOI: 10.1201/9781003741770-6 

significance of AI in gastroenterology has been increasingly acknowledged, leading to the inaugural global AI in gastroenterology and endoscopy summit held in Washington, DC, in late 2019. The summit convened numerous experts from academia, industry, and regulatory bodies. The consortium foresaw that within the next decade, the clinical integration of AI in gastroenterology would significantly impact patient care and streamline clinical workflows. Moreover, it emphasized the necessity of close multidisciplinary collaboration among gastroenterologists, industry stakeholders, and regulatory institutions for the development and implementation of new technologies in clinical practice [6].

Gastroenterology and hepatology involve the management of vast clinical data and a rich repository of imaging data from various sources like endoscopy, ultrasound, and computed tomography. Consequently, these fields are considered data-rich, providing fertile ground for AI applications. Extensive research has been conducted, particularly focusing on leveraging AI for the prevention, diagnosis, management, and prognosis of diseases within gastroenterology and hepatology [7, 8]. Our objective is to conduct a thorough review of AI applications in gastroenterology and hepatology, examining their breadth and depth. Simultaneously, we aim to pinpoint the present challenges in integrating AI into healthcare settings and explore potential solutions to address these obstacles.

## 6.2 GASTROENTEROLOGY

Gastroenterology is a field of healthcare dedicated to the identification and management of conditions impacting the digestive system, which encompasses the organs from the oral cavity to the anal opening along the digestive tract. This discipline handles a broad spectrum of issues related to the esophagus, stomach, small bowel, large bowel (colon), rectum, pancreas, gallbladder, bile ducts, and liver. In the following, an in-depth exploration of the various facets of gastroenterology is presented.

### 6.2.1 Anatomy and function

The gastrointestinal (GI) tract is an intricate network tasked with breaking down food, taking in nutrients, and eliminating waste. The process starts in the mouth and involves several organs, each with a specific function:

- Esophagus: Carries food from the mouth to the stomach.
- Stomach: Digests food by utilizing gastric juices.
- Small intestine: Further digests food and absorbs nutrients through its lining.

- Large intestine: Absorbs water and minerals, forming and storing feces.
- Liver: Produces bile for fat digestion, detoxifies harmful chemicals, metabolizes drugs, and processes nutrients.
- Gallbladder: Retains and intensifies bile produced by the liver, discharging it into the small intestine.
- Pancreas: Produces digestive enzymes and hormones, including insulin.

### 6.2.2 Common conditions

Gastroenterologists diagnose and treat a variety of diseases, such as:

- Gastroesophageal reflux disease (GERD): Acid reflux and heartburn due to stomach acid rising into the esophagus.
- Peptic ulcers: Open wounds or lesions that form on the inner surface of the stomach and the small intestine.
- Gastrointestinal inflammation disorders (GID): Encompasses Crohn's disease and ulcerative colitis, persistent ailments characterized by swelling and irritation in the digestive tract.
- Irritable bowel syndrome (IBS): A condition marked by a mix of stomach discomfort and changes in bowel movements.
- Gluten sensitivity disorder: A state where the immune system negatively responds to gluten intake, causing damage to the lining of the small intestine.
- Gallstones: Hard particles that form in the gallbladder or bile duct.
- Hepatitis: Inflammation of the liver, often caused by viruses, but also due to other factors like alcohol use.
- Pancreatitis: Inflammation of the pancreas.
- Colorectal cancer: Cancer of the colon or rectum, often detected through screenings like colonoscopies.

### 6.2.3 Diagnostic tools

Gastroenterologists use various tools and procedures to diagnose gastrointestinal diseases:

- Endoscopy: Including gastroscopy and colonoscopy, these procedures involve inserting a flexible tube with a camera into the GI tract.
- Ultrasound: Often used to visualize the gallbladder, liver, and pancreas.
- CT and MRI scans: Provide detailed images of the GI tract and surrounding structures.

- Biopsies: Removal of small tissue samples for examination under a microscope.
- Stool tests: Check for blood, infections, or markers of inflammation.

### 6.2.4 Treatment modalities

Treatment in gastroenterology may involve medication, lifestyle changes, or surgery:

- Medications: Can include antibiotics, anti-inflammatory drugs, acid blockers, and others depending on the condition.
- Diet and lifestyle changes: Often the first line of treatment for diseases like IBS or GERD.
- Surgical procedures: For more severe conditions, such as removing tumors or parts of the GI tract, correcting anatomical issues, or managing complications like bleeding.

### 6.2.5 Advanced research and techniques

Advancements in gastroenterology include the integration of AI for better diagnostic accuracy, personalized treatment plans, and management of complex cases. Research continues into the microbiome's role in GI health and diseases, and how modifying it can benefit conditions like Inflammatory Bowel Disease(IBD) and colon cancer. Gastroenterology remains a vital field in medicine due to the essential functions of the digestive system in overall health and the prevalence of GI diseases in the general population. It is a highly specialized field that requires comprehensive knowledge of the entire gastrointestinal system and its disorders. Figure 6.1 provides a comprehensive overview of gastroenterology.

## 6.3 ARTIFICIAL INTELLIGENCE

The domain of AI is a distinct branch of computational science dedicated to crafting frameworks that can carry out activities usually requiring human cognition. Such activities include acquiring knowledge, logical deduction, resolving challenges, sensory interpretation, and understanding linguistic patterns. These systems function through mathematical procedures, utilizing methodologies such as adaptive modeling, neural networking, and linguistic decoding. ML empowers AI to enhance its performance autonomously by analyzing extensive datasets and discerning patterns within them, without explicit programming. Deep learning, a subset of ML, employs neural networks comprising multiple layers to scrutinize various

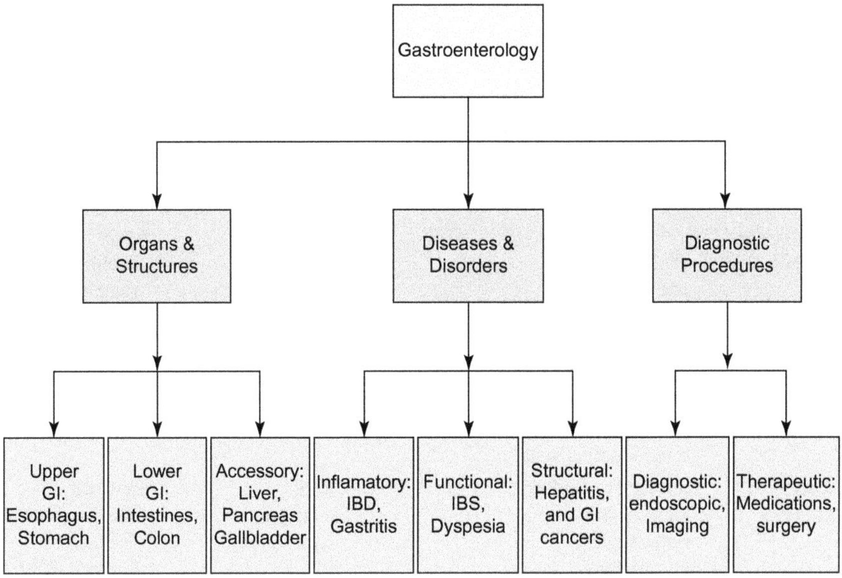


*Figure 6.1* Gastroenterology overview

data facets, thereby augmenting the system's proficiency in pattern recognition and decision-making.

## 6.4 ROLE OF AI IN GASTROENTEROLOGY

Machine learning and artificial intelligence-driven systems have been extensively utilized in the prediction, detection, handling, and outcome forecasting of digestive system disorders. These technologies address a wide array of conditions, ranging from digestive tract hemorrhages and bowel inflammation diseases to cancerous and precancerous growths, as well as other benign ailments like acid reflux, *Helicobacter pylori* (*H. pylori*) infestation, open sores in the stomach lining, gluten intolerance, and parasitic intestinal infections.

### 6.4.1 Prevention

Table 6.1 showcases the outcomes of research efforts utilizing AI and ML frameworks in the prevention of gastrointestinal disorders. These computational tools hold promise for use in early detection initiatives, identifying individuals at elevated risk outside of traditional criteria. In a recent study, scientists developed seven unique AI/ML algorithms aimed at isolating patients with an increased likelihood of developing stomach cancer

*Table 6.1* Prevention of gastroenterological diseases

| *Reference* | *Parameters* | *Classifier* | *Training/ validation set* | *Outcomes* |
|---|---|---|---|---|
| Leung et al. [9] | Findings from the lab, clinical, and pathological measures | Several | 64,238/25,330 patients | Danger of stomach malignancy emergence |
| Nakahira et al. [10] | Findings from the lab, clinical, and pathological measures, visuals from endoscopy | CNN | 7,826/454 patients | Assess the likelihood of gastric cancer emergence |
| Taninaga et al. [11] | Laboratory findings, clinical–pathological parameters, endoscopic visuals | CART | 1,186/292 | Prediction of future gastric cancer |
| Goshen et al. [12] | Laboratory findings, clinical, and pathological parameters | DT, RF, GB | 688 flagged patients | Elevated likelihood of Colorectal Cancer (CRC) progression |

following the elimination of *H. pylori* [9]. The advanced gradient boosting (GB) framework demonstrated exceptional efficacy. In another investigation, a DL architecture utilizing a CNN was developed to classify individuals into minimal, moderate, and elevated-risk categories for stomach cancer using endoscopy-derived visuals [10]. In a similar investigation, various decision trees for classification and regression (CART) were utilized to develop a predictive model estimating the probability of future gastric cancer occurrence. Another significant illustration is the ColonFlag test, a machine learning-based tool that leverages demographic factors such as age and gender, along with comprehensive blood count metrics, to detect individuals at heightened risk of colorectal cancer [11]. In a recent investigation that included 254 people who received a colonoscopy, scientists detected 19 instances of malignancy (7.5%) and 22 late-stage polyps (8.7%) among a group of patients who could have potentially skipped the diagnostic procedure [12]. These studies illustrate the practical application of AI/ML-based models in real clinical settings, particularly in establishing targeted screening programs.

### 6.4.2 Diagnostics

Table 6.2 provides a summary of the findings from selected research works that have utilized AI and ML algorithms for the detection of gastrointestinal disorders. These AI/ML-driven tools contribute to computer-assisted

*Table 6.2* Diagnose gastroenterological diseases

| *Reference* | *Diagnostic modality* | *AI classifier* | *Sizes of the training/validation sets* | *Outcomes* |
|---|---|---|---|---|
| Takiyama et al. [14] | Esophago-gastro-duodenoscopy imaging | CNN | 1,750/435 | Structural categorization within the voice box, food pipe, belly, and upper gut |
| Pace et al. [15] | Findings from the lab, clinical, and pathological measures | ANN | 195 patients | Identification of gastroesophageal reflux disease |
| de Groof et al. [16] | Esophageal endoscopic images | DNN | 1,285/295 | Classification of malignant from nondysplastic Barret's esophagus |
| van der Sommen et al. [17] | White-light endoscopy imaging | SVM | 48 individuals diagnosed with Barrett's esophagus | Identification of initial cancerous growths |
| Struyvenberg et al. [18] | Volumetric laser endomicroscopy imaging | Several | 65 individuals diagnosed with Barrett's esophagus | Diagnosis of neoplastic lesions |
| Swager et al. [19] | Volumetric laser endomicroscopy visualization | Several | 60 images | Identification of tumor growths |
| Kumagai et al. [20] | Endocytoscopic visualization | CNN | 4715/1520 | Detection of esophageal squamous cell carcinoma |
| Zheng et al. [21] | Endoscopic visuals | CNN | 1,545/458 patients | Identification of *H. pylori* infection |
| Nakashima et al. [22] | Endoscopic visuals | CNN | 162/60 patients | Identification of *H. pylori* infection |
| Itoh et al. [23] | Endoscopic visuals | CNN | 149/30 images | Identification of *H. pylori* infection |
| Kanesaka et al. [24] | NBI | SVM | 126/81 NBI images | Identification of stomach cancer |

detection or diagnosis (CAD) frameworks, which are commonly employed in radiology to improve the precision of analyzing medical scans. Generally, a CAD framework consists of initial data preparation, attribute identification, attribute refinement, and categorization phases.[13]. CAD systems could also support endoscopists in maneuvering through different areas of the gastrointestinal (GI) tract. Remarkably, a model based on CNN used images to precisely identify these anatomical sites, showcasing outstanding accuracy and effectiveness [14].

For diagnosing gastroesophageal reflux, an artificial neural network model was devised as a non-invasive diagnostic tool, solely utilizing clinical data [15]. A CAD system utilizing deep learning (DL) was tailored for patients diagnosed with Barrett's esophagus, with the goal of discerning between individuals with malignant conditions and those with nondysplastic Barrett's esophagus [16]. Additionally, the CAD system accurately pinpointed the optimal biopsy site, achieving an accuracy ranging between 92% and 97% [16]. In another study, a support vector machine (SVM) model was created utilizing white-light endoscopic imaging to detect early neoplastic lesions [17]. In a recent study, researchers used images captured through volumetric laser endomicroscopy to design a computer-based detection tool aimed at identifying precancerous lesions in people diagnosed with Barrett's esophagus [18]. A comparable investigation, which employed volumetric laser endomicroscopy, created a machine learning algorithm designed to identify cancerous growths [19]. Significantly, the model surpassed the performance of experts in volumetric laser endomicroscopy [19]. Ultimately, to identify esophageal squamous cell carcinoma, a CNN model was created, utilizing endocytoscopic images as an alternative to biopsy [20].

In a study focused on diagnosing patients with *H. pylori* infection, a CNN was developed using gastroscopic images [21]. In a preliminary pilot study, a unique convolutional neural network (CNN) for detecting *H. pylori* was created, examining visuals taken from the stomach's lesser curvature. These visuals were acquired through the use of either white light imaging, blue light imaging, or linked color imaging [22]. Substantially, the use of blue light and associated color imaging led to markedly better outcomes in comparison to white light imaging [22]. In a related study, a CNN model was employed to detect *H. pylori* infection using images captured during upper gastrointestinal (GI) endoscopy [23]. In the context of detecting gastric cancer, an SVM-driven computer-aided diagnosis system was developed to identify early signs of gastric cancer in narrow-band imaging (NBI) gastroscopy [24].

### 6.4.3 Treatment

The results of the studies that were found and used AI/ML models to treat gastroenterological disorders are compiled in Table 6.3. In a recent study,

*Table 6.3* Treatment of gastroenterological diseases

| *Reference* | *Parameters employed* | *AI classifier* | *Training/validation sets* | *Outcomes* |
|---|---|---|---|---|
| Rogers et al. [25] | Information from initial impedance, overnight initial impedance, and acid contact duration | DT | 335 patients | Forecasting treatment outcomes with proton-pump inhibitors for individuals suffering from gastroesophageal reflux disease. |
| Zhu et al. [26] | Endoscopic visuals | CNN | 780/212 images | Encroachment of stomach cancer into the mucosal and submucosal layers of the stomach. |
| Kubota et al. [27] | Endoscopic visuals | DNN | 790/80 images | Penetration level of stomach cancer. |
| Yamashita et al. [28] | Whole slide images (WSI) stained with hematoxylin and eosin | DNN | 100/15/484 | Recognition of CRC microsatellite instability. |
| Ichimasa et al. [29] | Experimental findings, clinical and pathological variables | SVM | 590/100 | Forecasting of the lymph node metastasis condition. |
| Levi et al. [30] | Experimental findings, clinical and pathological variables | RFE | 14,620 patients | Forecasting the requirement for blood transfusion after gastrointestinal bleeding (GIB). |
| Augustin et al. [31] | Experimental findings, clinical–pathological measures | CART | 164/103 patients | Layering of the likelihood of rebleeding and fatality after an acute variceal bleed. |
| Loftus et al. [32] | Findings from the lab, along with clinical and pathological indicators, were analyzed | ANN | 130/54 patients | Forecasting of critical lower gastrointestinal bleeding (GIB), anticipation of the necessity for operative intervention. |
| Ayaru et al. [33] | Laboratory results, clinicopathological parameters | GB | 180/110 | Forecasting of critical lower gastrointestinal bleeding (GIB), anticipation of repeated hemorrhage. |

a decision tree (DT) model was created to forecast the treatment outcomes for patients with gastroesophageal reflux disease (GERD) who are using proton-pump inhibitors. The model utilized data from baseline impedance, nocturnal baseline impedance, and acid exposure time [25].

Malignant gastrointestinal lesions have been managed using AI/ML-based models. In terms of stomach cancer, a CNN has been created to determine whether the early stage of the disease has spread to the stomach's mucosa and submucosa layers and to serve as a guide for endoscopic resection decisions [26]. Using the same idea, a Deep Neutral Network (DNN) was created to categorize stomach cancer according to invasion depth, which served as the foundation for therapy distribution [27]. In particular, T1, T1a, T1b, T2, T3, and T4 and an overall accuracy of 76.2%, 67.8%, 62.8%, 47.9%, 50.0%, 55.3%, and 63.8% were all successfully predicted by the model [27]. Finding microsatellite instability in colorectal cancer has a big influence on how treatments are distributed. To directly detect microsatellite instability from hematoxylin and eosin-stained samples, a DL model was created for the entire slide picture [28]. In order to determine whether patients would benefit from further therapy after the endoscopic removal of T1 tumors, an SVM model was created that predicted the lymph node metastatic status of patients with colorectal cancer [29]. To assess whether patients would gain advantages from additional treatment following the endoscopic excision of T1 tumors, an SVM model was developed to forecast the lymph node metastasis status in individuals with colorectal cancer [30]. In a study that focused on the lower Graph Information Bottleneck (GIB), two distinct ANN models were created with the goal of predicting the need for surgical intervention and severe acute lower GIB [32]. In a second study, a model based on a GB classifier was developed using nonendoscopic factors to predict the need for therapeutic intervention, recurrent bleeding, and severe lower GIB [33].

### 6.4.4 Prognosis

The results of the recognized studies using AI/ML models for the prognosis of gastroenterological disorders are compiled in Table 6.4. In a study, multiple SVM-based nomograms were created to forecast the likelihood of distant metastases in patients who underwent surgery for esophageal squamous cell carcinoma [34]. In another study, a neural network model was constructed using clinical and pathological data to forecast patient survival following curative surgery for esophageal cancer [35]. In order to predict recurrence in individuals who have had surgery for stomach cancer, a recent study created five distinct AI/ML-based models. The Random Forest (RF) model performed the best out of all the models [36].

An artificial neural network (ANN) model was created for IBD patients that utilized meteorological data to forecast seasonal differences in the

*Table 6.4* Prognosis of gastroenterological diseases

| *Reference* | *parameter* | *AI classifier* | *training/validation sets* | *Outcomes* |
|---|---|---|---|---|
| Yang et al. [34] | Experimental outcomes, immune indicators, clinical and pathological variables | SVM | 319/164 patients | Remote spread of esophageal squamous cell carcinoma post-operation. |
| Sato et al. [35] | Laboratory results, clinicopathological parameters, tumor characteristics | ANN | 398 patients (training: validation: test = 54:26:20) | Completely alter the 1-year and 5-year survival rates of individuals with esophageal cancer after surgical intervention. |
| Zhou et al. [36] | Experimental findings, clinical–pathological indicators, neoplasm features | Several | 2,054 patients (training: validation = 8:2) | Reoccurrence of stomach cancer after surgical intervention. |
| Peng et al. [37] | Meteorological data | ANN | 901 patients | Alterations in the commencement and recurrence of IBDs. |
| Hardalaç et al. [38] | Clinical and pathological characteristics, therapy information | ANN | 129 patients (training: validation: testing = 80:10:10) | Forecasting mucosal healing in CD patients receiving azathioprine treatment. |
| Takayama et al. [39] | Clinical and pathological characteristics, therapy information | ANN | 54/36 patients | Forecasting the necessity for surgery in UC patients undergoing cytoapheresis treatment. |
| Lyles et al. [40] | Findings from laboratory tests and clinical–pathological measures | CART | 875 patients | Forecasting in-hospital death risk for upper gastrointestinal bleeding (GIB) in patients with cirrhosis. |
| Grossi et al. [41] | Findings from laboratory tests and clinical–pathological measures | ANN | 815 patients | Fully change the 30-day mortality rate for non-variceal upper GIB patients. |
| Rotondano et al. [42] | Laboratory results, clinicopathological parameters | ANN | 2,380 patients | 30-day mortality of patients with non-variceal upper GIB. |

onset and relapse of CD and Ulcerative Colitis (UC) patients [37]. The model's mean absolute percentage error for the frequency of IBD beginning and relapse in the validation cohort was 37.58% and 17.1%, respectively [37]. An ANN model was created for CD research in order to forecast mucosal remission in patients receiving azathioprine 16 weeks after treatment [38]. An artificial neural network (ANN) was created in a UC study utilizing clinical data to predict which UC patients receiving cytoapheresis would eventually need surgery [39].

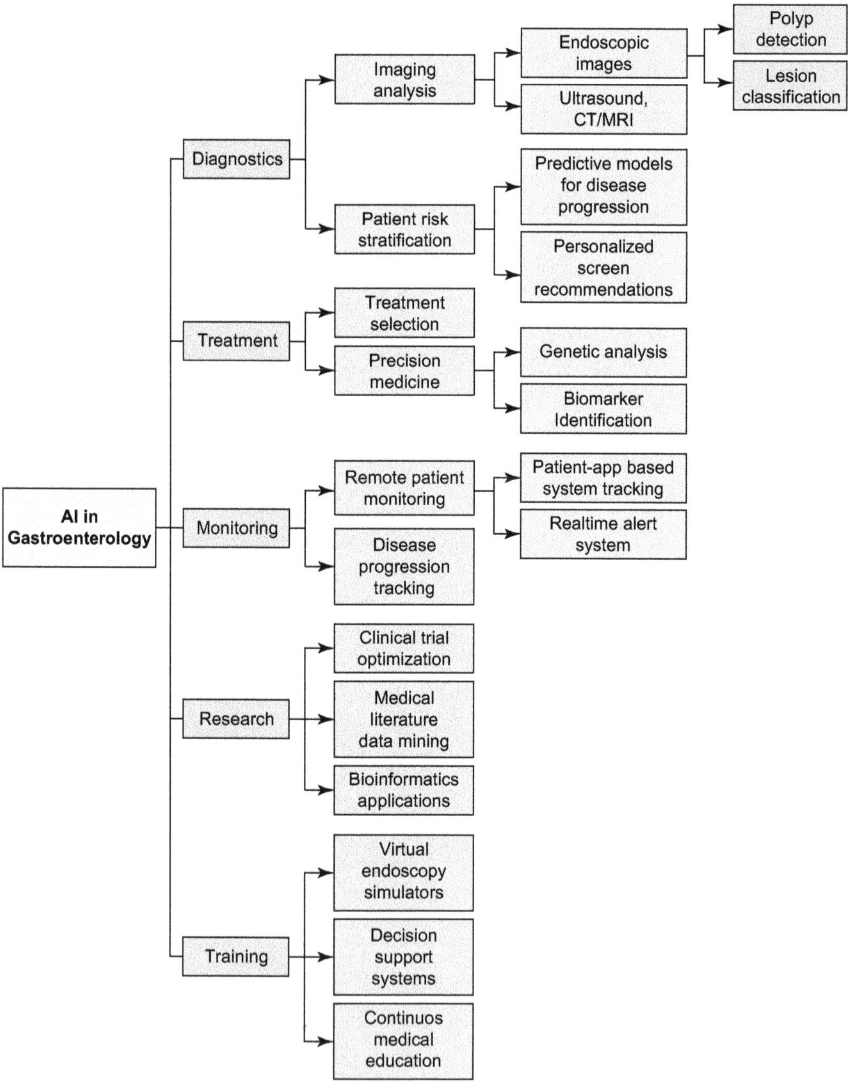


*Figure 6.2* Role of AI in gastroenterology

A CART model was created to forecast the in-hospital mortality of cirrhotic patients who come with upper GIB in relation to the prognosis of GIB [40]. An ANN model was created using pre-endoscopic characteristics in a multicenter trial to forecast 30-day mortality in patients with non-variceal upper GIB [41]. Similarly, pre-endoscopic factors were used in a prospective, multicentered investigation to create an ANN model that predicts 30-day mortality in patients with non-variceal upper GIB. Compared to the Rockall scoring method, the ANN fared substantially better (AUROCs: 0.95 vs 0.67) [42]. Figure 6.2 shows the role of AI in gastroenterology.

## 6.5 CHALLENGES

While the integration of AI into gastroenterology holds immense potential for advancing diagnostic accuracy, personalized treatment, and workflow efficiency, it also presents several challenges that hinder widespread adoption. These challenges stem from both technical and clinical aspects, such as data privacy, the interpretability of AI models, and integration within existing healthcare systems. Furthermore, concerns related to regulatory approvals, ethical considerations, and the need for large, high-quality datasets pose significant barriers. Some key challenges of AI in Gastroenterology are as follows:

- **Data privacy and security:** The sensitive nature of patient data in gastroenterology requires strict adherence to privacy regulations, such as Health Insurance Protability and Accountability Act (HIPAA). Ensuring data privacy while using AI tools can be challenging, especially with large-scale datasets.
- **Data availability and quality:** AI models require large, high-quality datasets for training. However, obtaining consistent, well-labeled, and annotated datasets in gastroenterology is difficult, leading to potential biases or inaccuracies in AI algorithms.
- **Lack of standardization:** There is limited standardization in the data formats, annotations, and protocols used across different gastroenterology practices, making it difficult to develop generalized AI models applicable across different clinical settings.
- **Interpretability of AI models:** Numerous AI systems, particularly deep learning models, operate as "opaque entities," complicating clinicians' ability to understand the reasoning behind their decisions. This absence of clarity can erode confidence among healthcare professionals.
- **Integration into clinical workflow:** Incorporating AI tools into existing gastroenterological practices can be challenging due to workflow

disruptions, requiring significant adjustments in routine clinical procedures and staff retraining.

- **Regulatory challenges:** The regulatory approval process for AI tools in healthcare is still evolving. Obtaining approval for AI systems, especially those used in decision-making in gastroenterology, is complex due to the need for clinical validation.
- **Ethical considerations:** AI systems can unintentionally reinforce biases inherent in the training data, resulting in disparate impacts on various patient groups. Addressing ethical concerns, such as equity, bias reduction, and patient consent, is a significant challenge.
- **Cost and resource constraints:** Implementing AI technologies in gastroenterology requires significant financial investment, from acquiring data infrastructure to training staff. This can be a barrier, particularly for smaller practices.
- **Lack of skilled workforce:** There is a shortage of healthcare professionals with both medical and AI expertise, which is critical for developing and validating AI systems tailored for gastroenterology.
- **Continuous learning and adaptability:** AI models in gastroenterology must be continually updated to accommodate new medical knowledge and adapt to evolving clinical guidelines. Keeping these systems up-to-date requires ongoing monitoring and retraining.
- **Liability and accountability:** Determining responsibility when AI systems fail or make incorrect decisions is a significant legal and ethical challenge. It is unclear whether clinicians, AI developers, or healthcare institutions should be held accountable.

## 6.6 CONCLUSION

As AI continues to evolve, its applications in gastroenterology are becoming increasingly promising. AI has the ability to enhance diagnostic accuracy, streamline workflows, and support decision-making processes in various aspects of gastroenterology, including endoscopy, imaging, and disease management. By utilizing extensive datasets and sophisticated algorithms, AI can assist in recognizing patterns that might be difficult for humans to discern, enhancing early detection and leading to better patient outcomes. In conclusion, AI has great potential to improve many areas of gastroenterology, from diagnosing diseases to personalizing treatments and improving patient care. However, numerous obstacles remain that must be tackled before its complete incorporation into clinical settings. These include ensuring data privacy, creating high-quality datasets, overcoming regulatory hurdles, and making AI tools easier for doctors to understand and use. With continued research and collaboration between medical and AI experts, AI could become a valuable tool in advancing the field of gastroenterology and improving patient outcomes.

## REFERENCES


1. Noorbakhsh-Sabet, Nariman, et al. "Artificial intelligence transforms the future of health care." *The American Journal of Medicine* 132.7 (2019): 795–801.
2. Calderaro, Julien, and Jakob Nikolas Kather. "Artificial intelligence-based pathology for gastrointestinal and hepatobiliary cancers." *Gut* 70.6 (2021): 1183–1193.
3. Hoogenboom, Sanne A., Ulas Bagci, and Michael B. Wallace. "Artificial intelligence in gastroenterology. The current state of play and the potential. How will it affect our practice and when?" *Techniques and Innovations in Gastrointestinal Endoscopy* 22.2 (2020): 42–47.
4. Deo, Rahul C. "Machine learning in medicine." *Circulation* 132.20 (2015): 1920–1930.
5. Wu, Jia, Jiamin Chen, and Jianting Cai. "Application of artificial intelligence in gastrointestinal endoscopy." *Journal of Clinical Gastroenterology* 55.2 (2021): 110–120.
6. Parasa, Sravanthi, et al. "Proceedings from the first global artificial intelligence in gastroenterology and endoscopy summit." *Gastrointestinal Endoscopy* 92.4 (2020): 938–945.
7. Le Berre, Catherine, et al. "Application of artificial intelligence to gastroenterology and hepatology." *Gastroenterology* 158.1 (2020): 76–94.
8. Yang, Young Joo, and Chang Seok Bang. "Application of artificial intelligence in gastroenterology." *World Journal of Gastroenterology* 25.14 (2019): 1666.
9. Leung, Wai K., et al. "Applications of machine learning models in the prediction of gastric cancer risk in patients after Helicobacter pylori eradication." *Alimentary Pharmacology & Therapeutics* 53.8 (2021): 864–872.
10. Nakahira, Hiroko, et al. "Stratification of gastric cancer risk using a deep neural network." *JGH Open* 4.3 (2020): 466–471.
11. Kinar, Yaron, et al. "Development and validation of a predictive model for detection of colorectal cancer in primary care by analysis of complete blood counts: A binational retrospective study." *Journal of the American Medical Informatics Association* 23.5 (2016): 879–890.
12. Goshen, Ran, et al. "Computer-assisted flagging of individuals at high risk of colorectal cancer in a large health maintenance organization using the ColonFlag test." *JCO Clinical Cancer Informatics* 2 (2018): 1–8.
13. Mosquera-Lopez, Clara, et al. "Computer-aided prostate cancer diagnosis from digitized histopathology: a review on texture-based systems." *IEEE Reviews in Biomedical Engineering* 8 (2014): 98–113.
14. Takiyama, Hirotoshi, et al. "Automatic anatomical classification of esophagogastroduodenoscopy images using deep convolutional neural networks." *Scientific Reports* 8.1 (2018): 7497.
15. Pace, Fabio, et al. "Artificial neural networks are able to recognize gastro-oesophageal reflux disease patients solely on the basis of clinical data." *European Journal of Gastroenterology & Hepatology* 17.6 (2005): 605–610.
16. de Groof, Albert J., et al. "Deep-learning system detects neoplasia in patients with Barrett's esophagus with higher accuracy than endoscopists in a multistep training and validation study with benchmarking." *Gastroenterology* 158.4 (2020): 915–929.

17. van der Sommen, Fons, et al. "Computer-aided detection of early neoplastic lesions in Barrett's esophagus." *Endoscopy* 48.07 (2016): 617–624.
18. Struyvenberg, M. R., et al. "Improved Barrett's neoplasia detection using computer-assisted multiframe analysis of volumetric laser endomicroscopy." *Diseases of the Esophagus* 33.2 (2020): doz065.
19. Swager, Anne-Fré, et al. "Computer-aided detection of early Barrett's neoplasia using volumetric laser endomicroscopy." *Gastrointestinal Endoscopy* 86.5 (2017): 839–846.
20. Kumagai, Youichi, et al. "Diagnosis using deep-learning artificial intelligence based on the endocytoscopic observation of the esophagus." *Esophagus* 16 (2019): 180–187.
21. Zheng, Wenfang, et al. "High accuracy of convolutional neural network for evaluation of Helicobacter pylori infection based on endoscopic images: preliminary experience." *Clinical and Translational Gastroenterology* 10.12 (2019): e00109.
22. Nakashima, Hirotaka, et al. "Artificial intelligence diagnosis of Helicobacter pylori infection using blue laser imaging-bright and linked color imaging: a single-center prospective study." *Annals of Gastroenterology* 31.4 (2018): 462.
23. Itoh, Takumi, et al. "Deep learning analyzes Helicobacter pylori infection by upper gastrointestinal endoscopy images." *Endoscopy International Open* 6.02 (2018): E139–E144.
24. Kanesaka, Takashi, et al. "Computer-aided diagnosis for identifying and delineating early gastric cancers in magnifying narrow-band imaging." *Gastrointestinal Endoscopy* 87.5 (2018): 1339–1344.
25. Rogers, Benjamin, et al. "Artificial intelligence automates and augments baseline impedance measurements from pH-impedance studies in gastroesophageal reflux disease." *Journal of Gastroenterology* 56 (2021): 34–41.
26. Zhu, Yan, et al. "Application of convolutional neural network in the diagnosis of the invasion depth of gastric cancer based on conventional endoscopy." *Gastrointestinal Endoscopy* 89.4 (2019): 806–815.
27. Kubota, Keisuke, et al. "Medical image analysis: computer-aided diagnosis of gastric cancer invasion on endoscopic images." *Surgical Endoscopy* 26 (2012): 1485–1489.
28. Yamashita, Rikiya, et al. "Deep learning model for the prediction of microsatellite instability in colorectal cancer: a diagnostic study." *The Lancet Oncology* 22.1 (2021): 132–141.
29. Ichimasa, Katsuro, et al. "Artificial intelligence may help in predicting the need for additional surgery after endoscopic resection of T1 colorectal cancer." *Endoscopy* 50.03 (2018): 230–240.
30. Levi, Riccardo, et al. "Artificial intelligence-based prediction of transfusion in the intensive care unit in patients with gastrointestinal bleeding." *BMJ Health & Care Informatics* 28.1 (2021).
31. Augustin, Salvador, et al. "Predicting early mortality after acute variceal hemorrhage based on classification and regression tree analysis." *Clinical Gastroenterology and Hepatology* 7.12 (2009): 1347–1354.
32. Loftus, Tyler J., et al. "Neural network prediction of severe lower intestinal bleeding and the need for surgical intervention." *Journal of Surgical Research* 212 (2017): 42–47.

33. Ayaru, Lakshmana, et al. "Prediction of outcome in acute lower gastrointestinal bleeding using gradient boosting." *PLoS One* 10.7 (2015): e0132485.
34. Yang, H. X., et al. "Support vector machine-based nomogram predicts postoperative distant metastasis for patients with oesophageal squamous cell carcinoma." *British Journal of Cancer* 109.5 (2013): 1109–1116.
35. Sato, Fumiaki, et al. "Prediction of survival in patients with esophageal carcinoma using artificial neural networks." *Cancer: Interdisciplinary International Journal of the American Cancer Society* 103.8 (2005): 1596–1605.
36. Zhou, Chengmao, et al. "A machine learning-based predictor for the identification of the recurrence of patients with gastric cancer after operation." *Scientific Reports* 11.1 (2021): 1571.
37. Peng, Jiang Chen, Zhi Hua Ran, and Jun Shen. "Seasonal variation in onset and relapse of IBD and a model to predict the frequency of onset, relapse, and severity of IBD based on artificial neural network." *International Journal of Colorectal Disease* 30 (2015): 1267–1273.
38. Hardalaç, Fırat, et al. "The rate of mucosal healing by azathioprine therapy and prediction by artificial systems." *Turkish Journal of Gastroenterology* 26.4 (2015): 315–321.
39. Takayama, Tetsuro, et al. "Computer-aided prediction of long-term prognosis of patients with ulcerative colitis after cytoapheresis therapy." *PLoS One* 10.6 (2015): e0131197.
40. Lyles, Thomas, Alan Elliott, and Don C. Rockey. "A risk scoring system to predict in-hospital mortality in patients with cirrhosis presenting with upper gastrointestinal bleeding." *Journal of Clinical Gastroenterology* 48.8 (2014): 712–720.
41. Grossi, Enzo, et al. "Artificial neural networks for early prediction of mortality in patients with non-variceal upper GI bleeding (UGIB)." *Biomedical Informatics Insights* 1 (2008): BII-S814.
42. Rotondano, Gianluca, et al. "Artificial neural networks accurately predict mortality in patients with nonvariceal upper GI bleeding." *Gastrointestinal Endoscopy* 73.2 (2011): 218–226.

Chapter 7

# Artificial intelligence in drug delivery

*Ira Singh, Santosh Kumar, Joonseok Koh, and Abilio J.F.N. Sobral*

## 7.1 INTRODUCTION

The creation of novel medicinal delivery methods with maximum efficacy and low adverse effects has garnered increasing attention in recent decades [1–3]. Both controlled drug administration and the limitations of traditional drug delivery methods, such as systemic toxicity, narrow therapeutic index, and challenges in dose adjustment during prolonged treatment, have been well researched [2, 3]. Developing implantable microchips with microfabrication technologies appears to be a viable strategy for precise medication delivery [4]. Microfabricated drug delivery systems enable continuous or pulsatile release of medication through drug reservoirs of varying capacities and geometries, which can be activated on demand [5]. These multifunctional and highly sophisticated devices for controlled drug release have addressed many of the challenges associated with traditional delivery systems [6]. Considerations like dose modification, targeted distribution, sustained release, and intelligent control systems are necessary for designing implantable drug delivery systems [7]. Control systems have been developed utilizing neural networks (NN), fuzzy logic, integrators, and differentiators [8]. Among drug delivery techniques are microrobots, micro-pump mechanisms, and focused ultrasound [9]. A promising method for medication delivery is the creation of micro- or nanoparticles using microfluidic systems [10]. Innovative drug delivery systems, including Janus micro- or nanoparticles that can disperse several drugs, are made possible by the application of microfluidic technology [11]. A microchip implant by Microchips, Inc., combines wireless communication technologies, integrated electronic components, and a power source to dispense medication in a regulated manner. The pulsating release lasted for around half a year [12]. An initial clinical trial has employed implantable microchips for medicine delivery in osteoporotic patients [13]. Controlled insulin administration combined with ongoing glucose monitoring may greatly lessen the difficulties associated with diabetes. Integration of the insulin delivery system, glucose sensors, control algorithms, and mathematical models is useful in this situation. For the administration of insulin and glucose monitoring, an automated

 DOI: 10.1201/9781003741770-7

system that integrates the insulin pump, dose calculator, and glucose meter into a single device has been developed [3, 14], targeting distribution, drug stability, and consideration of elements such as medicine release rates and on-demand dosage modifications while developing intelligent administration systems [15]. Well-designed algorithms are required to be used with self-monitoring delivery devices to regulate the quantity and timing of drug release [3]. Smart drug delivery systems are being developed using artificial neural networks (ANNs), wireless communication, and information technology. These systems may be able to overcome the drawbacks of traditional treatment approaches [2, 3]. Devices for regulated drug distribution have greater versatility thanks to wireless connections. The devices give data to the monitors, receive orders from outside sources, and control the flow of drugs [3]. Software that models pharmacodynamics and pharmacokinetics, simulates biological processes, generates control algorithms, delivers drugs under controlled conditions, and evaluates the effectiveness of treatment plans has been developed using biologically inspired computing models, composed of interconnected processing units that simulate a network of model neurons [3, 16, 17]. The application of machine learning (ML) methods to ligand-based target prediction has given rise to the concept of target fishing (TF), a technique that identifies protein targets of new biologically active compounds by leveraging ligand databases, target proteins, and the interactions between ligands and their respective targets [18, 19]. The use of cutting-edge technology is essential for the development of novel delivery procedures and the upcoming generation of medications. This chapter emphasizes the pivotal impact of AI on the formulation of drug delivery strategies and explores the intricate challenges associated with their development.

## 7.2 THE FUNDAMENTALS OF ARTIFICIAL INTELLIGENCE (AI)

### 7.2.1 Tracing the growing role of AI in healthcare

In the 1960s and 1970s, Dentrals saw the development of the first problem-solving software with applications in organic chemistry in mind. Microcomputers gained popularity in the 1980s and 1990s, and new degrees of network connectivity were added. Researchers and developers realized at this time that artificial intelligence systems used in healthcare had to be built to account for the lack of artificial neural networks, which were previously used in intelligent computing systems. Artificial intelligence's uses in the healthcare industry have grown, thanks to developments in technology and medicine during the past 50 years. Natural language processing, genetic expansion, adoption of an electronic health record system, increased volume and accessibility of health-related data, improvements in computing power, and robot-assisted surgery can all make it possible [20]. Research on artificial intelligence has increased across a number of medical specialties in recent years. One of the greatest uses of artificial intelligence is to promote health and reduce the need for medical care—or at least to a minimum. Applications of artificial intelligence in consumer health and the internet of medical things are already helping people. Technology-driven applications encourage people to adopt healthier behaviors and support the proactive maintenance of a healthy lifestyle. Customers have control over their health thanks to it [21]. Diseases like cancer can now be identified earlier and more accurately thanks to artificial intelligence. The American Cancer Society states that a significant percentage of mammograms result in false positives, which may cause mistakes. Reviewing and translating mammograms 30 times more quickly and accurately is now feasible because of artificial intelligence [22]. The area of radiology in particular has drawn the most attention. Clinicians may find it easier to notice a subtle alteration in a picture that they might otherwise overlook if they can evaluate imaging results. Microsoft's Hanover Project analyzes medical research to determine which cancer drug treatment option will be most beneficial for patients. It is affiliated with Oregon Health and Science University's Knight Cancer Institute. Other efforts involve the creation of programmable cells and the processing of medical images to track the progression of tumors. The UK National Health Service is using data gathered from a mobile app to identify specific health risks using the Google DeepMind platform. In a second initiative with the NHS, computer vision algorithms to identify malignant tumors are developed by analyzing medical images obtained from NHS patients. The corporation's venture capital division, Intel Capital, has made an investment in Luminata, a business that develops treatment plans and identifies high-risk patients using artificial intelligence (AI) [23].

By examining data fragments kept in the cloud, a distributed memory system, any artificial intelligence digital equipment, can feel and detect objects, understand and react to recognized signals, form opinions, and even learn to change its views and behaviors. The development of artificial intelligence in the healthcare industry is seen in Figure 7.1. The invention of turning tests in 1950 was the first significant application of AI in medicine. The importance of AI in healthcare was first acknowledged in 1975 with the National Institutes of Health (NIH) hosting the first central artificial intelligence in medicine (AIM) symposium and creating the first medical computer research facility. With the introduction of DeepQA and the advancement of deep learning (DL) in the 2000s, artificial intelligence has become more prevalent in the healthcare industry. Furthermore, the first pharmacy robot wasn't made until 2015, but the cardiac assist device (CAD) was initially utilized for endoscopy in 2010. In 2017, as artificial intelligence entered the medical domain, the Food and Drug Administration (FDA) released the first cloud-based DL application that had received

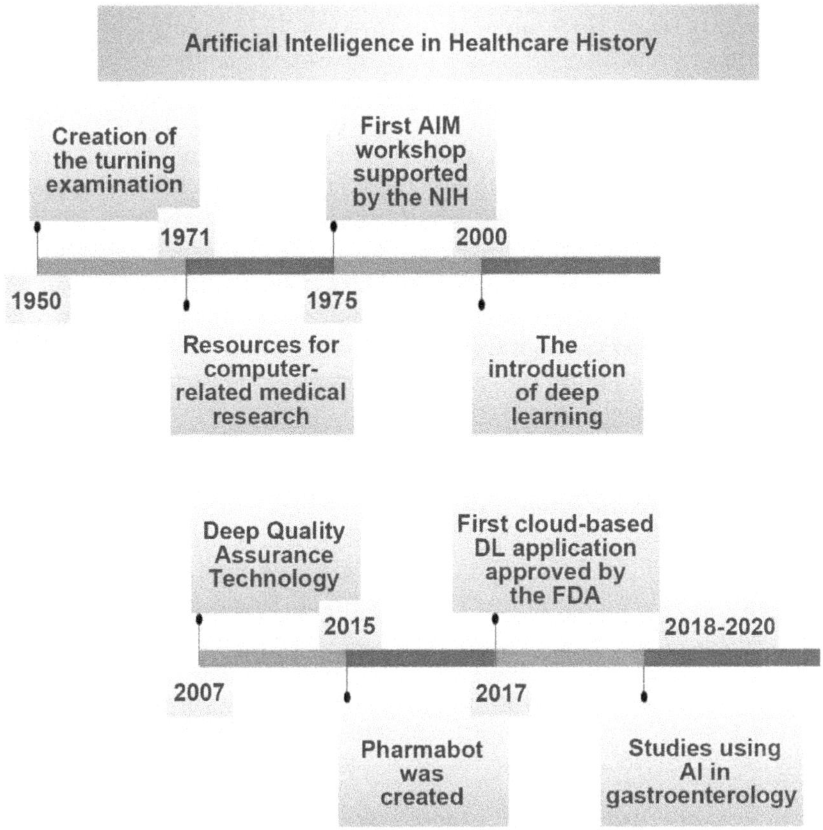


*Figure 7.1* Timeline illustrating the evolution of artificial intelligence in healthcare

approval. Between 2018 and 2020, a large number of AI experiments in gastroenterology were carried out [24].

### 7.2.2 Harnessing AI across medicine and the pharmaceutical industry

Unlike other conventional healthcare technologies, artificial intelligence technology can gather data, process it, and provide end users with a clearly defined result [25]. Machine learning algorithms are used by artificial intelligence to do this. Complex algorithms are solved by artificial intelligence, and software is utilized to assess human intelligence when analyzing intricate medical data. The capacity of computer algorithms to generate educated estimates without direct human input is known as artificial intelligence. Algorithms are able to recognize patterns in behavior and produce their own logic. Repeated testing is necessary to lower the mistakes in the output of artificial intelligence. Algorithms used in artificial intelligence function differently from humans; for example, once an objective is determined, they cannot change on their own; instead, they can only comprehend precise instructions. It is difficult to read about healthcare in the future and not understand it fully. Since the field of artificial intelligence research was founded in 1956, very little progress has been achieved in improving medical practice. Real life and the hype surrounding machine learning started to collide [26]. The delivery of healthcare benefits greatly from artificial intelligence. Artificial intelligence has been used in therapeutic settings far more frequently in recent years. Artificial intelligence systems come in useful with their ability to mine data and identify patterns, especially when it comes to treating or managing diseases. Modern medicine faces a huge difficulty in gathering, interpreting, and utilizing organized and unstructured data. Artificial intelligence in medicine can aid with disease management, diagnosis, and prognosis [27]. Artificial intelligence applications in medicine use illness symbols and analyze their relationship to patient symptoms and indicators. In addition to drug development, patient monitoring, and treatment protocol development, diagnostic artificial intelligence programs collect, aggregate, and compare clinical data with predefined illness classifications to aid in diagnosis and therapy [28]. Figure 7.2 illustrates how artificial intelligence has five significant applications in the healthcare and pharmaceutical industries that totally change the game. Among these uses are clinical development, research discoveries, supply chain management, manufacturing, monitoring of patients, and post-market surveillance [24].

### 7.2.3 Categories of artificial intelligence

Healthcare firms can now evaluate a wide range of data thanks to artificial intelligence, machine learning, and DL. They provide increasingly deeper insights that result in proactive treatment, less risk in the future, and optimized workflow. Artificial intelligence, machine learning, and DL all refer to various aspects of machine learning, even though DL is a subset of machine learning. Machine learning and related technologies are included in the wide idea of artificial intelligence. Understanding how the technologies work together is essential [29].

#### *7.2.3.1 ML*

The purpose of computational models is to achieve artificial intelligence ideas within the machine learning subset. The algorithms self-adapt and change to perform better in the future whenever they gradually come into contact with new information. As machines examine data, they are actually learning. This process enables artificial intelligence algorithms to choose tasks that have the best possibility of succeeding. Biometric scanning

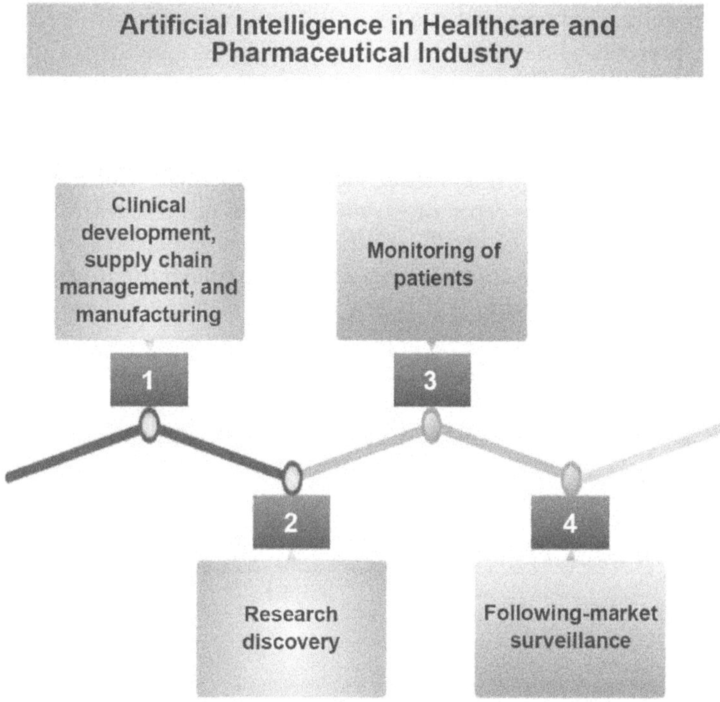


*Figure 7.2* Diverse applications of artificial intelligence across the healthcare and pharmaceutical industries

and medical claims tend to be just two instances of the data sources that machine learning uses [23].

### 7.2.3.2 DL

This finds patterns in the data by employing several network layers, including abstract layers created by human engineers. With the use of this technology, unstructured data may be given structure and robots can be taught to independently classify data. As the use of robotics in spine surgery grows, more research is being done on the accuracy of the technology, its ability to reduce intraoperative radiation, and its overall surgical efficiency. According to a study, 379 orthopedic patients found that using robotic technology aided by artificial intelligence (called Mazor Robotics) minimized surgical complications five times more often than using free-hand doctors. The first robotically assisted retinal surgery experiment was successfully completed by Oxford. Twelve individuals in need of retinal dissection were randomized to receive surgery with a robot or by hand while under general anesthesia. In the groups that had manual and robotic surgery, artificial intelligence yielded the longest surgical results. The market for artificial intelligence is still developing, best practices are being defined, and successful technology adoption presents some difficulties. They have to take security and patient privacy into account. The costs of developing, maintaining, and repairing emerging technology are typically surpassed by long-term expenditures in intelligent technologies. Organizations can reap numerous advantages by embracing the future of intelligence, such as expedited and precise diagnosis, decreased human error rates, and reduced administrative expenses [23]. The classification of artificial intelligence is displayed in Figure 7.3. Russell and Norvig have created seven kinds of artificial intelligence in their book *Artificial Intelligence: A Modern Approach*. Among these are robotics: Motion and manipulation, logic and issue-solving, natural language processing, planning and social intelligence, vision, machine learning, and knowledge representation. Three important subcategories of machine learning are supervised learning, unsupervised learning, and deep learning.

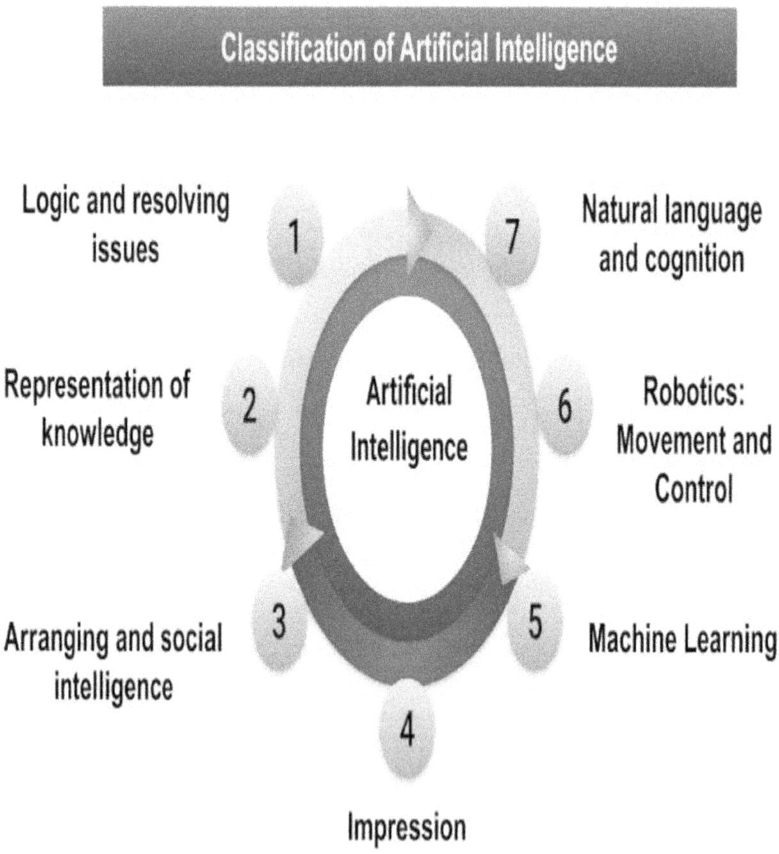


*Figure 7.3* Classification of artificial intelligence

Machine vision and image recognition are two subcategories of vision, on the other hand. Just as the natural language, classification, machine translation, question answering, text generation, and content extraction are the five primary areas of processing. Speech technology is further subdivided into two major categories: Text-to-speech and speech-to-text [24].

### 7.2.4 Key foundations and tools of AI and ML

In the following, the most commonly used machine learning models in drug delivery and treatment research are presented.

#### *7.2.4.1 Boost*

One type of group learning called Boost aims to increase the resilience of the prediction by training numerous models with the same structure. To provide a set of alternative models, ensemble learning trains a large number of models whose parameters are initialized at random. To minimize noise, bias, and volatility, the final forecast integrates the projections from these multiple models. Boost strategy may frequently increase precision and dependability when compared to a single model. Several boosting techniques have been developed, including adaptive boosting (AdaBoost) [29], gradient tree boosting (GTB) [30], extreme gradient boosting (XGBoost) [31], and categorical boosting (CatBoost) [32]. By continuously merging multiple weak machine learning models into a single, powerful model, AdaBoost enhances performance. To regulate the importance of the training data, it gives each weak model learnable weights; the weights of the accurately identified samples drop with each iteration while those of mistakenly identified samples increase. As a result, the weak model in the subsequent iteration concentrates on the misclassified data with the highest weights. Each sample point's gradient direction and associated residuals are decreased in order to train the GTB ensemble of decision trees. Following the same gradient boosting concepts, XGBoost avoids overfitting by optimizing the function's aim, the tree's size, and the weights' magnitude. CatBoost, a variant of the gradient boosting method, might manage category information without leaking targets.

#### *7.2.4.2 Decision trees and random forest*

One kind of rule-based machine learning method is decision trees [33]. One illustration of a chain is a decision tree that looks like a tree. It generally comprises a root node representing the complete training dataset, several branch nodes denoting decision points, and multiple leaf nodes that reflect the final outcomes of those decisions. The data is divided into homogeneous subsets by each branch node using a unique set of splitting rules. Until a particular requirement is satisfied (for example, how many depth samples exceed the specified maximum value) or until every sample inside the subsets has the same label, the data will be divided into progressively smaller subsets. The most commonly used decision tree algorithms, based on different splitting criteria, include ID3 [34], C4.5 [35], and the Classification and Regression Tree (CART) [36] algorithm. The "randomt" [37] (ML) is a collection of decision trees that makes up the model constructed by using the bagging technique. It's short for bootstrap aggregating, is specifically designed for random forests, and works by combining the predictions of multiple tree models—each typically overfitted, high in variance, and low in bias—into a unified and more reliable prediction set. Random forest can improve the machine learning model's overall performance by aggregating the predictions from multiple decision trees [38].

#### 7.2.4.3 *Support vector machine (SVM)*

SVM is a powerful machine learning model that uses kernels to find subtle patterns in complex datasets [39]. A higher-dimensional latent space can be created from the original low-dimensional input feature space, where the data are not linearly separable, by employing the "kernel trick" in support vector machines. The following is the mathematical conclusion of the SVM:

$$y(x) = w1\varphi(x1) + w2\varphi(x2) + \ldots + wn\varphi(xn) + b$$

However, the weights and bias derived from the training data are contained in the W = [w1, w2, ..., wn]. The b$\varphi$ kernel function can be Gaussian, linear (without kernel), or a comparable radical basis function (RBF). The support vectors are sampled at the decision Wb boundary and determine the weight and bias. The SVM training process selects the parameter weight and bias to split the training samples linearly, $\Phi$, in order to maximize the margin of the high-dimensional latent space supplied by the kernel function.

Nonetheless, selecting the appropriate kernel function has an impact on SVM performance, and selecting the optimal kernel for a given recognition task is not predetermined. Actually, the best-performing kernel is chosen using the validation data set [39].

#### 7.2.4.4 *k-nearest neighbors (kNN)*

In 1967, Cover and Hart presented kNN [40]. It is an instance-based approach that necessitates the storage of every training sample. One may rapidly ascertain a test sample's prediction by looking at the connection between the test individual and the examples kept in the instructional data. kNN is resilient against data noise and is simple to implement. It can function effectively on tiny datasets that possess an equal number of samples that are positive and negative [41].

#### 7.2.4.5 Logistic regression

The ML model known as logistic regression (LR) is often used for binary categorization since its parameters are simple to comprehend. Its ability to discriminate enables it to function effectively [42]. One popular machine learning method for evaluating clinical data in the medical field is logistic regression [43]. The likelihood that a sample will fall into a class is calculated using a linear approach. The discriminative model known as logistic regression ignores the input and output joint distribution and then maps the input feature vector to the output to directly calculate the posterior probability.

The linear relationship between log changes and attributes [44], which is one of the limitations of logistic regression, is typically not met when attempting to illustrate the link between exposure and response in infectious diseases, such as human immunodeficiency virus (HIV) [45].

#### 7.2.4.6 Artificial neural networks

Artificial neurons, which are linked together and are thought to be the fundamental information processing units, make up ANNs [46]. Neural networks, which resemble the neurons in the human brain, are another name for ANNs. The fundamental structural elements of an ANN are neurons. The following is a representation of each neuron:

$$z(x) = f(w1x1 + w2x2 + \ldots wnxn + b)$$

where f is the activation function (often the sigmoid function); in DL, the rectified linear unit and z(x) is the neuron's output given the input x. Backpropagation is used to learn the parameters of weights and W = [w1, w2, ..., wn], bias b from the training set of data [47]. By modeling the input–output mappings that are not linear, the human brain served as the inspiration for the nonlinear mathematical model known as the neuron. An artificial neural network (ANN) typically consisting of a minimum of three layers is involved: (1) An input layer that receives data by allocating a value to each feature to a neuron; (2) one or more hidden layers that use weighted linear combinations to process and transmit information; and (3) an output layer that generates the final result, frequently with a nonlinear activation function to add complexity and enhance intelligence. To be more precise, every layer comprises several neurons, each of which is linked to every other neuron in the layer below it to transfer data between the input and the output [46].

#### 7.2.4.7 *Set covering machine (SCM)*

SCM is an ML technique that creates unusually sparse rule-based models by taking a greedy approach [48]. It might identify the logical pairings of Boolean-valued rules—like conjunction, logical-AND, or disjunction, logical-OR—that are produced from the data. For instance, based on whether or not a genetic trait is present in a genome, rules can predict a phenotype [48]. SCM has the sparsity property, which means that domain experts may understand its predictions with fewer rules because it is a sparse model that can produce output with a small collection of features. This is because SCM predictions are based on simple Boolean-valued rules [48].

#### 7.2.4.8 *Feedback system control (FSC)*

By means of the differential evolution (DE) search method, the FSC closed-loop search algorithm looks for the best possible combinations of the input variables. It is appropriate for usage in numerous applications [49]. The fundamental tenet of FSC is that it only considers system feedback or the variations between the anticipated and actual system responses. The DE search method finds the best combinations or iteratively evolves the system towards a desired result [50, 51], using the feedback as the optimization criteria.

#### 7.2.4.9 *NB*

Naïve Bayes (NB) is a biomedical informatics model that has been used since 1961. It is a straightforward, incredibly powerful machine learning model that excels at multi-class prediction [52]. Because it is an interpretable model, it is feasible to ascertain how each feature affects the final prediction [53]. Nevertheless, the fundamental premise of naïve Bayes is that every feature ought to be autonomous, which isn't true for real data. Furthermore, the posterior probabilities are nearly always 0 or 1. When working with data that has big feature vector dimensions, its performance is limited [54]. Table 7.1 highlights the key characteristics of the machine learning models discussed, emphasizing the distinct advantages each provides in real-world data applications.

## 7.3 INTEGRATION OF ARTIFICIAL INTELLIGENCE WITH NANOTECHNOLOGY (NT)

### 7.3.1 Combining artificial intelligence with nanotechnology

Overall, AI and NT have an impact on several scientific fields and may result in the development of smarter gadgets [55]. The combination of AI

*Table 7.1* A succinct summary of the key features of machine learning techniques commonly applied in drug delivery

| *Machine learning techniques* | *Benefit(s)* |
|---|---|
| Boost | – Increase accuracy and dependability.<br>– CatBoost may handle category information without causing target leakage [32]. |
| Decision trees and random forest | – To improve the machine learning model's overall performance, aggregate the predictions from multiple decision trees [38].<br>– The bagging technique is specifically made for random forests [38]. |
| Support vector machine (SVM) | – Identify minute patterns in complicated datasets [39].<br>– Using variable kernels based on structural risk minimization and model nonlinearity. |
| k-nearest neighbors (kNN) | – Is resilient against data noise and is simple to implement [41].<br>– It can function effectively on tiny datasets that possess an equal number of samples that are positive and negative [41]. |
| Logistic regression | – Its parameters are easily interpreted [42].<br>– Its capacity for discrimination allows it to deliver high-quality performance [42]. |
| Artificial neural networks (ANN) | – Several input variables are included in the data model.<br>– No presumption of independence among the inputs. |
| Set covering machine (SCM) | – Demonstrates the logical combinations of Boolean-valued rules—such as conjunction, disjunction, logical-AND, and logical-OR—that are generated from the data [48].<br>– Easy to comprehend and interpret. |
| Feedback system control (FSC) | – Driven by output.<br>– It is appropriate for usage in numerous applications [49]. |
| Naïve Bayes | – Straightforward and incredibly effective machine learning model [52].<br>– Works well in multi-class prediction [52]. |

and nanotechnology (NT) will be advantageous to these domains (Figure 7.4), resulting in more individualized, successful, and efficient drug delivery strategies. Techniques from artificial intelligence (AI) have been used to address issues in nanotechnology, including those related to nanoscale simulation, nanosystem design, and nanocomputing (AI) methods that can be applied to interpretation of experimental data, new design concepts, quicker calculation speeds, and effective parameter estimates and system modeling [55]. The physical limitations of nanotechnology could be overcome by artificial intelligence (AI) paradigms, which could produce nanoarchitectures with more computational power [56]. AI paradigms and techniques are helpful for creating simple simulations at the nanoscale and for developing nanodevices, such as nanocomputers, that can do complicated tasks, including processing sensory data [55]. Machine learning

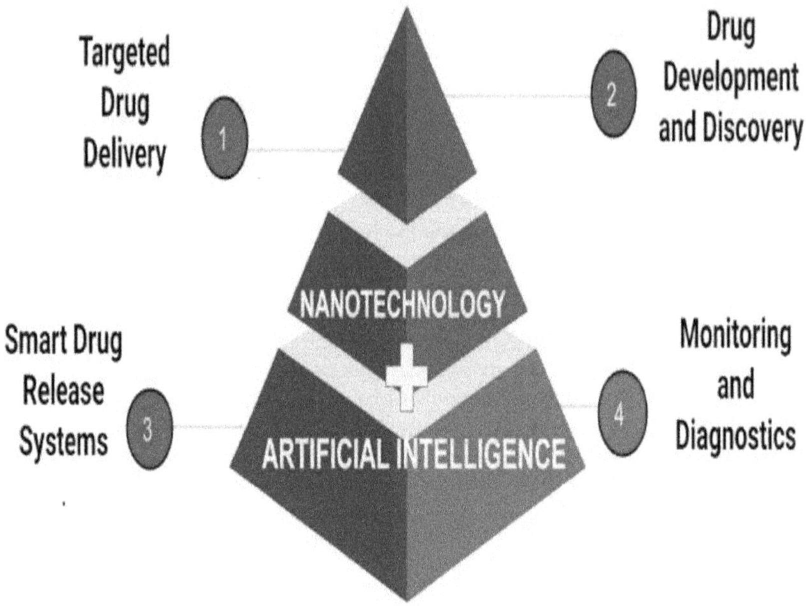


*Figure 7.4* Five areas of drug delivery where the combination of AI and nanotechnology will have a big impact

paradigms are implemented by nanocomputing devices, including bio-inspired ones [57], which may be crucial for resolving challenging analytical issues. Developing chemical libraries, finding new drug candidates with ideal qualities, forecasting the roles of proteins in biology, and DL are all essential components of contemporary drug development [58]. Therapeutic development in biopharmaceutical businesses may be more successful if AI systems are used for biological data analysis, therapeutic target identification, and pharmaceutical search [59]. Finding new medications or targets may depend on the ability to predict target–drug interactions using machine learning approaches [60]. There is a proposed regularized least squares classifier as an effective supervised learning technique for drug–target interaction prediction [60]. Furthermore, when it comes to predicting drug–target interactions, the semi-supervised link prediction classifier has demonstrated exceptional effectiveness [61]. Least squares regularization and Gaussian interaction profiling kernels both perform well in terms of prediction; however, the predictive capacity is enhanced when Gaussian interaction profile, chemical, and genomic kernels are mixed together [62]. The top ANN-based models have shown good performance across a range of experimental methodologies when compared to experimental data [63]. Forecasting the pharmacological characteristics of medications, including their modes of action and indications, is now possible thanks to deep neural network models [58]. Furthermore, drug metabolism is modeled by machine learning techniques, which can lead to more precise predictions of the potential toxicity and metabolic outcomes of new medication options. These models contain links between drug chemical structures and biological outcomes, interactions between medications and metabolic enzymes, and metabolic endpoints [64].

### 7.3.2 How nanomedicine can be revolutionized by artificial intelligence

Combinatorial nanomedicine's recent developments have produced the perfect environment for AI-driven optimization. For example, co-delivery of multiple nanoparticle types has significantly enhanced tumor targeting and treatment efficacy. Specifically, the first application of gold nanoparticles was for localization at tumor locations. Next, doxorubicin-loaded liposomes covered in a protein called Factor XIII analogue, which facilitates fibrin crosslinking during coagulation, were given as a second class of nanoparticles. The clotting process significantly enhanced this complex's binding sites, which raised drug localization at the tumor site by a factor of 40 and significantly increased therapeutic efficacy [65]. The co-administration of irinotecan-loaded multifunctional mesoporous silica nanoparticles (MSNPs), also known as silicasomes, and iRGD, a tumor-penetrating peptide, is another instance of co-delivery to improve tumor penetration. By attaching to the NRP-1 receptor and initiating a nutrient transport pathway, cyclic tumor-penetrating peptide-unconjugated iRGD promotes the transcytosis of carrier silicasomes. Extremely aggressive tumors called pancreatic ductal adenocarcinoma (PDAC) have demonstrated a threefold to fourfold increase in silicasome absorption when paired with iRGD. Improved treatment results resulted from this, including a decrease in metastases and an increase in total survival time [66]. Poly(lactic acid-*co*-glycolic acid)–polyethylene glycol (PLGA–PEG) nanoparticles containing and co-localizing two different kinds of treatments, siRNA and cisplatin prodrug, illustrate how well nanoparticles may stabilize and distribute synergistic combinations. The route of translesion DNA synthesis (TLS) expression is restricted by siRNA, siREV1, and siREV3L working together. Although chemotherapy-induced DNA damage can be repaired by tumor cells thanks to this unstable process, it also raises the possibility that the cells will become resistant to the treatment. PLGA–PEG nanoparticles for the simultaneous administration of siREV1, siREV3L, and a cisplatin prodrug effectively supported siRNA-mediated suppression of TLS activity, which is associated with acquired mutagenic drug resistance. This approach was demonstrated in mouse models to prevent additional tumor growth and increase overall survival while also enhancing cellular sensitivity to the cytotoxic cisplatin's regulated release [67]. Additionally, medicines that work in concert with other forms of treatment can be administered with the help of nanoparticles. Multifunctional up-conversion core/porous silica shell nanotheranostics (UCSNs), for example, consist of a core composed of dual-functional up-conversion nanoparticles (UCNPs) encapsulated with cisplatin, which has been demonstrated to clinically enhance radiotherapy, and an outer shell composed of a porous silica layer for accurate magnetic imaging targeting. It has been displayed that UCSNs can target cancers using luminescence/magnetism dual-mode imaging and may efficiently administer cisplatin to tumors for a combination of radiation and chemotherapy [68].

Combining artificial intelligence with medication delivery based on nanotechnology can lead to notable improvements in treatment outcomes, even though combination therapy tactics based on nanomedicine have increased treatment efficacy. It has been shown that when several drugs are given using nanotechnology platforms, they cooperate to target several disease pathways. This is because combo treatment based on nanomedicine has the same limitations as combination therapy that has not been altered, meaning that variations in drug synergy resulting from patient heterogeneity may pose a threat to fixed-dose, multi-drug delivery. In a new investigation, four drugs—unmodified paclitaxel, nanodiamond-doxorubicin, nanodiamond-bleomycin, and nanodiamond-mitoxantrone—were used in combination therapy, and artificial intelligence was used to optimize the drug–dose ratios globally. Several control cell lines (IMR-90, H9C2, MCF-10A) and several breast cancer cell lines (MDA-MB-231, MCF-7, BT20) were analyzed at the same time. The goal of the investigation was to optimize and determine the best concentrations of the medication combinations to achieve maximum control cell line survival and maximum cancer cell killing. Phenotypic response surfaces from the Latin hypercube sampling mode experiment could be utilized to rapidly identify the optimal dosages. This study is significant because it shows that AI-optimized drug combinations for nanomedicine performed better than AI-enhanced unaltered medication combinations, unaltered and nanomedicine-altered monotherapies, and randomly generated nanomedicine combinations. The study's optimization objective was to determine the best concentrations of the medication combinations to achieve maximum control cell line survival and maximum cancer cell killing. Furthermore, it was demonstrated that most of these unplanned combinations of nanomedicines were more harmful than helpful. It's interesting to remember that bleomycin, mitoxantrone, and doxorubicin are comparable treatments. According to conventional drug development, these drugs would combine to produce a compounding effect. This investigation, however, demonstrated that finding the ideal drug–dose ratios significantly increased efficacy above and beyond an additive effect. This illustrated how important dose optimization is when designing combo therapies [69].

Important considerations to make while creating a sophisticated nanomedicine include targeting, localization effectiveness, release profiles, and other aspects of nanodrug composition. However, since all of these elements work together to determine treatment success, AI can directly optimize for it and it has an extremely enticing feature: its optimization procedures implicitly account for these qualities. As such, they are taken into consideration when the optimization process is put into practice.

### 7.3.3 AI-powered drug delivery nanorobots

The primary components of nanorobots are integrated circuits, sensors, a power source, and a safe data backup; computational technologies like artificial intelligence (AI) keep them up to date [70]. Among their abilities are target identification, collision avoidance, sensing and attaching, and ultimately leaving human anatomy. Nano/microrobots' ability to move through target locations, depending on addressing physical aspects, for instance pH, has increased their effectiveness and reduced their detrimental systemic effects [71]. Considerations such as dose adjustment, sustained release, and control release must be made while developing implanted nanorobots for the regulated delivery of drugs and genes. Additionally, AI methods like NNs, uncertain reasoning, and integrators must be used to automate the medication release [72]. Microchip-based prosthetics can be used for both body position detection and programmed release.

## 7.4 APPLICATION OF AI APPROACHES TO DIFFERENT BIOLOGICAL SYSTEMS FOR DRUG DELIVERY SYSTEMS

### 7.4.1 Insulin delivery

The three primary types of diabetes are type 1 diabetes, type 2 diabetes, and gestational diabetes according to research. One characteristic that distinguishes type 1 diabetes is hyperglycemia or high blood glucose. The user can get insulin via a syringe, insulin pen, or insulin pump, among other options. Subcutaneous injection, however, is commonly utilized because of its benefits, which include high absorption capacity, affordability, and effective administration. Patients may experience pain and infections if injections are administered frequently. Hypoglycemia from suboptimal insulin supply can lead to brain damage, coma, behavioral and cognitive abnormalities, and even death. As a result, scientists have been studying several insulin delivery methods, including transdermal, nasal, and non-invasive delivery as well as controlled dosing [73]. A common autoimmune disease, type 1 diabetes, primarily damages the beta islet cells of the pancreas. It can result in insulin insufficiency and elevated blood sugar levels in the host [74, 75]. Pancreatic implantation or islet replacement is one of the most popular standard treatments for diabetic patients to manage their decreased beta-cell function. Unfortunately, no ideal method for providing enough functional beta-cells has been developed due to resource constraints. Consequently, closed-loop control delivery is the ideal choice for diabetes individuals. Figure 7.5 illustrates the fundamental closed-loop insulin therapy system for blood glucose regulation.

Since 1950, numerous researchers have been examining closed-loop drug delivery devices. In 1980, Miles Laboratories' BIOSTATARTM system—a device that uses insulin infusion to help diabetics control their blood glucose levels—became the first to be approved for premarket use [76]. These days, the closed-loop artificial pancreas is among the highest promising advancements in effective diabetes treatments; however, validations are still being conducted [77]. An appropriate system, an insulin infusion pump, and glucose monitoring capabilities could potentially be included in the fully automated, closed-loop artificial pancreas as technology develops [78]. For closed-loop control, a number of control strategies have been effectively

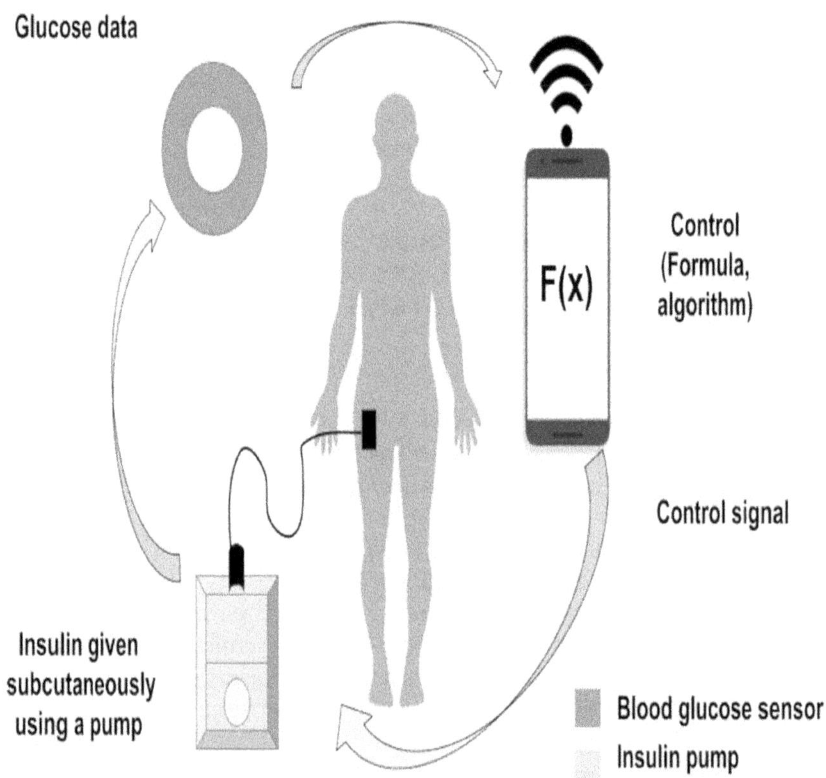


*Figure 7.5* An elementary block schematic of an insulin delivery

established, including traditional PID [79], H-infinity [80], model predictive control (MPC) method [81], Sliding Mode Control (SMC) [82], fuzzy logic control (FLC) [83], and neural networks [84]. Dudde and Vering looked into the automated delivery of insulin using an MPC technique [81]. Kaveh and Shtessel proposed SMC as a means of regulating diabetics' blood glucose readings [85]. Utilizing an H-infinity controller, the management of a type 1 diabetic patient's blood glucose levels was illustrated by Yasini et al. [86]. Using a control technique with patient-specific model-predictive control, a customized scheduling strategy, a state estimator, and an open-loop optimization formulation connected to patient-specified process models and constraints, Zavitsanou et al. examined a personalized optimal insulin delivery [87]. The suggested adaptive control technique's performance and robustness were evaluated against the traditional zone MPC strategy utilizing the FDA-approved UVA/Padova simulator with a cohort of 100 adults [88]. Furthermore, Shi et al. suggested a control penalty adaptation technique for zone model predictive control (MPC) in artificial pancreas systems based on the anticipated glucose levels and their rate of change [89]. Only clinical use was permitted for the first MiniMed closed-loop glucose monitoring device to be sold commercially. Three days' worth of data from the download and analysis of blood glucose levels were recorded by this subcutaneous device [90]. The FDA authorized MiniMed® 670G for commercial use in 2017, enabling closed-loop basal glucose management through the use of a wearable insulin pump and a closed-loop glucose sensor. The only tasks required for the user of the currently available device, which functions as a closed-loop hybrid system, require manual meal boluses, food and activity data submission, and sensor data calibration two to four times daily. Thus, the need for a completely closed-loop system continues to be a topic of discussion among scientists and academics. Companies such as Abbott, Bigfoot Biomedical, Dexcom, Tandem Diabetes Care, Senseonics, and Roche have recently adopted collaborative strategies to jointly explore and advance closed-loop systems in the coming years [90].

As a result, control engineers and other scientists continue to struggle with the creation of insulin therapy's closed-loop control system. Additional technical requirements for closed-loop systems, like insulin pumps, may include reduced dimensions, enhanced safety features, and sufficient energy efficiency. Additional advancements in closed-loop glucose monitoring may involve optimizing algorithms and reducing the size of glucose sensors to increase patient comfort or enable long-term implantability.

### 7.4.2 Drug delivery in cardiac ailments

Although the field of cardiac assist devices (CAD) has made tremendous strides, the application of control systems and modeling principles is relatively new [91]. According to Elnaggar et al. [92], various control strategies have been developed for cardiac pacemaker design, including adaptive PID control, fuzzy logic-based PID techniques, and fuzzy logic control (FLC) methods. Additionally, Shi looked at a fuzzy PID-based intelligent control strategy for cardiac pacemakers. For people with heart problems, a crucial first step is the identification of heart disease. Consequently, one option to exercise stress testing is pharmacological stress testing. In order to diagnose CAD, a drug–device closed-loop system was created. Signs of ischemia resulted from an intravenous infusion of the catecholamine arbutamine, which raised heart rate and cardiac contractility [93]. The average arterial blood pressure is another important aspect of the cardiac system that has changed recently due to developments in control theory (MABP). It is among the human body's most important hemodynamic parameters because postoperative hypertension may lead to serious outcomes like hemorrhage, vascular suture line rupture, and cerebrovascular accidents. In a range of clinical contexts, including the delivery of anesthesia, cardiac surgery, and the postoperative recovery phase, it should stay within stable parameters [94]. For the automated control of mean arterial blood pressure (MABP) during drug infusion, a number of control mechanisms have been put forth over time. These consist of neural networks [95], fuzzy logic control (FLC) [96], model predictive control (MPC) [97], fractional order control [98], PID controllers, adaptive controllers [99], model reference adaptive control [100], robust multiple model adaptive control [51], and reinforcement learning [101]. Kwok and colleagues displayed medication delivery via a computer method that uses silica nanoparticle (SNP) infusion to automatically regulate MABP. The control method incorporates optimization terms with both finite and infinite horizons, and one of its components is long-range predictive control. Recursive control relevant identification is used by the control algorithm to operate adaptively in the suggested long-range predictive control strategy [102]. In 1992, Ying et al. [97] examined a closed-loop control for SNP drug infusion-based MABP regulation in postoperative patients using a fuzzy-PI controller. An evolving vague rule with several inputs emulation network system and its learning mechanism was created by Treesatayapun for computerized supervision of MABP for the distribution of injectable SNP medications [104]. Polycarpou and Conway developed an adaptive (NN) approach for modeling and closed-loop regulation of MABP by referencing an adaptive monitoring using a passive model for SNP treatment flow [103]. Gao and Er presented an extended fuzzy neural network-based adaptive control and modeling approach for blood pressure management by SNP injection. A linear feedback control method was used to apply the feedforward generalized neural network [105]. Prior to its removal from the market in 2012, the IVAC titrator (IVAC Corporation, based in San Diego, California, USA) was the only commercially available device, according to Doyle et al. [106]. The FDA had only authorized the IVAC titrator system as an SNP in an enclosed loop medication delivery mechanism for reducing blood pressure after cardiovascular surgeries before its premarket release [107]. It was withdrawn from the market due to several factors, including outdated computer interface technology, a lack of trustworthy communication standards at the time, a difficult-to-use customized blood pressure sensor, a high price tag, and an unknown impact on patient outcomes due to reduced variability. However, with improved microprocessor-based pump technologies and new communication standards, an industry boost could come from an MABP closed-loop network [106].

Furthermore, there is a great chance to dominate the market with dependable and reasonably priced automated blood pressure systems—including implantable devices—that can enhance patients' quality of life and lessen the workload for physicians and caregivers in the current era of the Internet of Things (IoT), wireless technologies, AI-driven control strategies, and micro-electro-mechanical systems (MEMS) advancements. A closed-loop control system for cardiac therapy using ingestible drugs is depicted in a block diagram form in Figure 7.6.

### 7.4.3 Targeted drug delivery for gastrointestinal tract disorders

The gastrointestinal system of the body is involved in conditions like Crohn's disease, small intestine tumors, and cryptic gastrointestinal disorders. The tailored administration of dosages is necessary for the treatment of certain chronic illnesses. A specific location along the gastrointestinal tract receives a constant dose of drug through controlled drug delivery devices [108]. These days, more research is being done on gastrointestinal system medicine administration that is both dependable and focused. The wireless capsule endoscope is one tool that might be utilized to diagnose and treat illnesses related to the gastrointestinal (GI) tract [109]. Over the past few years, numerous writers have been attempting to create an effective endoscopy in capsule (CE) examining Israel's imaging in Yoqneam [110]. Since the standard endoscope was unable to reach the whole gastrointestinal tract, the M2A capsule endoscope was created in 2000 and utilized to examine the small intestine. This CE is powered by peristalsis and has a light source, video imager, transmitter, and batteries all housed in a tiny 11 × 26 $cm^3$ plastic cylindrical container [111]. Despite a number of developments, wireless CE was mostly utilized for diagnostic purposes; as a result, there was significant worry over the usage of CE for treating GI tract illnesses. Thus, a number of researchers created several cutting-edge tools for delivering drugs locally. These tools are called InteliSite (Innovative Devices LLC), Enterion capsule (Phaeton Research), and IntelliCap by Philips Electronics. Because of the peristaltic movement, the medication would spread throughout a small area of the lumen, and the delivery mechanisms

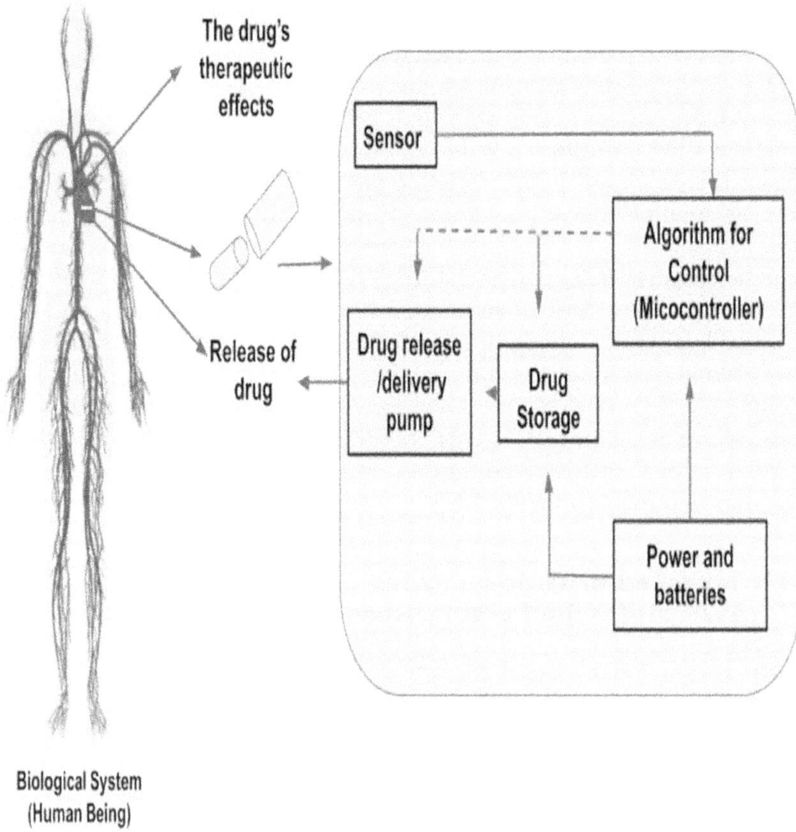


*Figure 7.6* Block schematic showing a closed-loop medication administration system intended for heart problems

of these devices are unable to target the particular pathogen. They lack a way to halt the activity and maintain a specific posture [112]. According to Li et al., a clip-releasing mechanism was used to create the first purpose of the endoscope for therapeutic cordless capsules, for the treatment of gastrointestinal bleeding [113].

Medimetrics and Philips created IntelliCap®, the first smart, electronic, oral capsule intended for targeted, minimally invasive medicine delivery in the gastrointestinal tract. It features integrated technology, including temperature and pH sensors, along with wireless radio frequency communication capabilities. A personal computer is used to control it and distribute customized medications at a specified time and location [114]. Along the same lines, Le et al. (2016) presented a medication delivery module made of soft magnet materials that developed features including drug release and placement control using active locomotive intestinal capsule endoscopy [115]. Leung et al. looked at a therapeutic method for treating gastrointestinal hemorrhage that used a balloon tamponade effect. Applying pressure between the lesion and the GI wall, the inflatable balloon was employed to stop the bleeding in the GI tract [116]. Since oral drug administration is advised, swallowable tablets are becoming more and more popular because of their low cost and high patient acceptance [117]. Smart tablets are helpful in managing gastrointestinal disorders such as irritable bowel syndrome, gastroesophageal reflux, and esophageal cancer as well as locally activated diseases [118]. Devices for capsule endoscopy feature coin batteries, data transfer, and cameras built right in. Previously, these endoscopic pills moved by means of the GI tract's natural peristalsis motion, which had drawbacks such as the inability to stop and regulate the risk of capsule retention in the tract. As a result, numerous researchers have been attempting to provide the endoscope capsule with a mode of mobility. Figure 7.7 illustrates a

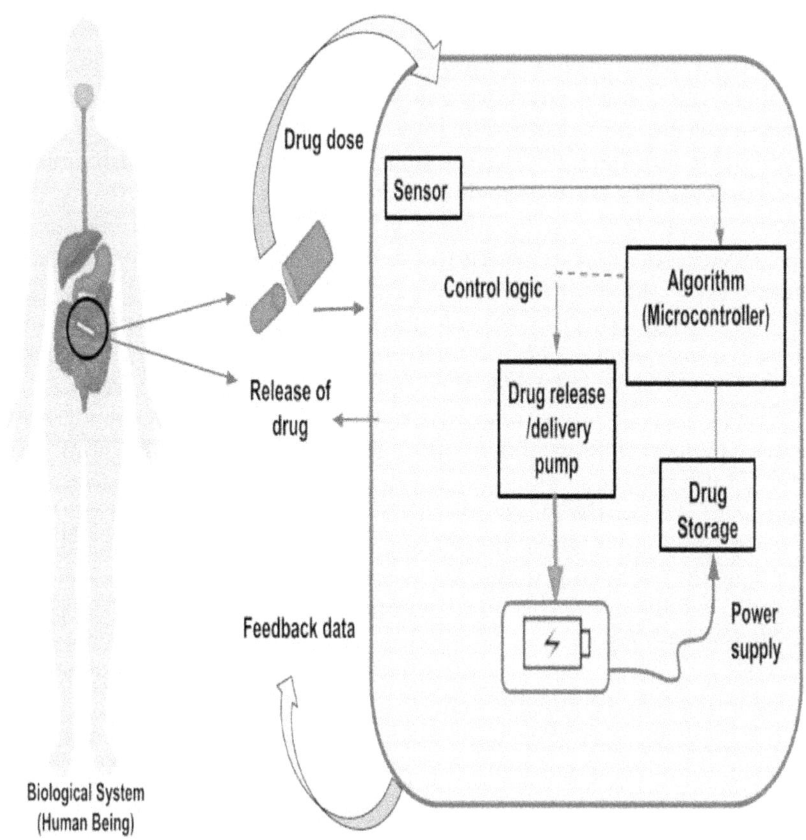


*Figure 7.7* A basic block diagram illustrating a swallowable drug-based, closed-loop control system for addressing gastrointestinal tract issues

basic closed-loop drug administration method employing swallowable pills or capsules for GI tract problems. In 2019, Luo et al. prepared an AI-driven diagnostic system for the gastrointestinal tract to analyze clinical endoscopic images and provide a tool for detecting gastrointestinal cancer [119]. In 2020, Sofer et al. presented advanced learning methods for percutaneous cordless pill and offered a comprehensive, methodical examination of the approach's implementation [120].

Recent advancements in closed-loop treatment systems for gastrointestinal disorders have centered on developing efficient actuators and incorporating advanced AI-driven control strategies. These innovations present numerous opportunities for the near future.

### 7.4.4 Drug delivery for cancer treatments

Nowadays, cancer has become a global concern for scientists, engineers, and medical professionals. Tumors, which are aberrant cell growths that are out of control and unregulated, are included in the category of cancer. If treatment for these tumors is delayed, they have the potential to spread to other body parts, assault the surrounding tissues, and finally result in the patient's death. The most prevalent type of cancer is brought on by both internal and environmental factors, including immunological disorders, tobacco use, poor food, and mutations [121]. Tumor development results from an imbalance between apoptosis and cell growth. Furthermore, the rate at which these malignant cells proliferate is exponential. When this cell imbalance persists for a long time and is treated inappropriately, cancer cells proliferate unchecked, ultimately leading to cancer patients' deaths [122]. Numerous methods such as immunotherapy, hormone treatment, chemotherapy, radiation treatment, surgery, or a mix of these are available for treating cancer. Chemotherapy is the method of treating cancer patients that is most frequently employed among these. After the treatment session is over, eliminating the aberrant cancer cells is a crucial goal of the chemotherapy strategy [123]. Yet, the right course of action, including chemotherapeutic drugs, which can only kill tumor cells, has not yet been found [124].

Figure 7.8 illustrates the fundamental approach for closed-loop delivery of chemotherapeutic agents in clinical trial settings. Furthermore, the closed-loop delivery of drugs used to treat cancer would be adequately controlled by AI-based control systems.

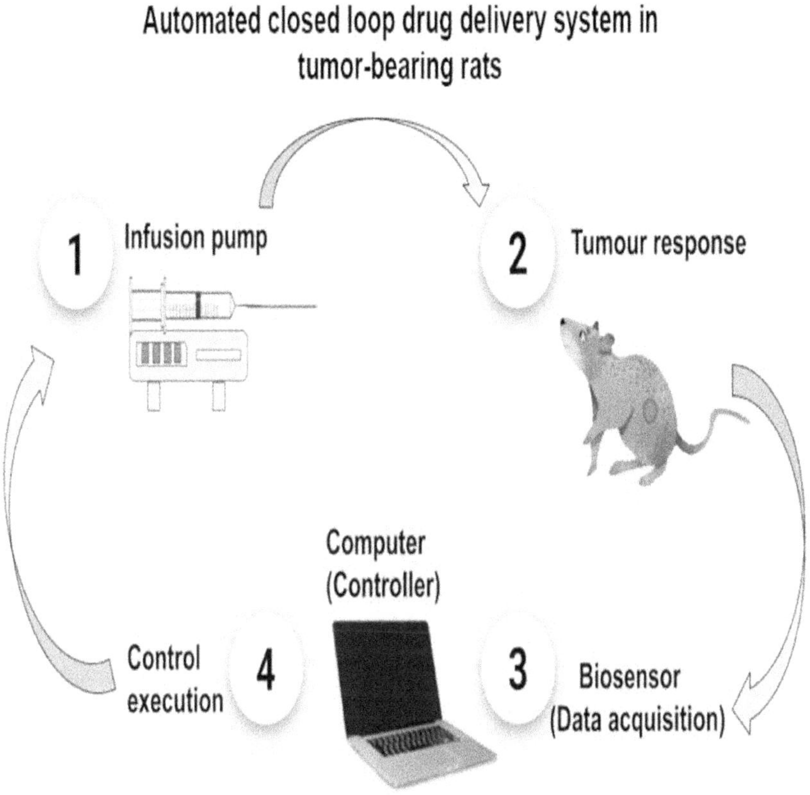


*Figure 7.8* The fundamental framework of an automated drug delivery system with closed-loop control for cancer treatment

## 7.5 CONCLUSION

Artificial intelligence could fundamentally transform drug delivery in the future. It is possible to significantly increase the accuracy, effectiveness, and safety of drug administration by utilizing AI technologies. AI-driven techniques enable personalized medicine, where treatment regimens are tailored to each patient's particular profile, maximizing therapeutic results and minimizing side effects. Concerns including data privacy, ethical quandaries, and the need for comprehensive clinical validation persist despite the positive advancements. Future research should focus on resolving these problems and enhancing AI systems in order to increase their anticipated accuracy and robustness. AI's ongoing development in drug delivery holds out the possibility of opening doors for more efficient and patient-focused healthcare solutions, which will eventually improve health and quality of life for people all over the world.

## LIST OF ABBREVIATIONS

| | |
|---|---|
| AdaBoost | Adaptive Boosting |
| AI | Artificial Intelligence |
| ANN | Artificial Neural Networks |
| CART | Classification and Regression Tree |
| CatBoost | Categorical Boosting |
| DL | Deep Learning |
| DNA | DeoxyriboNucleic Acid |
| FDA | Food and Drug Administration |
| FSC | Feedback System Control |
| HIV | Human Immunodeficiency Virus |
| GTB | Gradient Tree Boosting |
| IoT | Internet of Things |
| kNN | k-Nearest Neighbors |
| MABP | Mean Arterial Blood Pressure |
| MCF-7 | Michigan Cancer Foundation-7 |
| ML | Machine Learning |
| PLGA–PEG | Poly(Lactic acid-*co*-Glycolic Acid)–PolyEthylene Glycol |
| SCM | Set Covering Machine |
| SVM | Support Vector Machine |
| TNBC | Triple-Negative Breast Cancer |
| TF | Target Fishing |
| XGBoost | Extreme Gradient Boosting |

## REFERENCES

1. P. Tangri and S. Khurana, "Pulsatile drug delivery systems: methods and advances," *International Journal of Drug Formulation and Research*, vol. 2, 2011, pp. 100–111.
2. A. Maroni, L. Zema, M. D. Del Curto, G. Loreti, and A. Gazzaniga, "Oral pulsatile delivery: Rationale and chronopharmaceutical formulations," *International Journal of Pharmaceutics*, vol. 398, no. 1–2, 2010, pp. 1–8.
3. M. Staples, K. Daniel, M. J. Cima, and R. Langer, "Application of micro-and nano-electromechanical devices to drug delivery," *Pharmaceutical Research*, vol. 23, 2006, pp. 847–863.
4. K. B. Sutradhar and C. D. Sumi, "Implantable microchip: the futuristic controlled drug delivery system," *Drug Delivery*, vol. 23, no. 1, 2016, pp. 1–11.
5. J. T. Santini Jr A. C. Richards, R. Scheidt, M. J. Cima, and R. Langer, "Microchips as controlled drug-delivery devices," *Angewandte Chemie International Edition*, vol. 39, no. 14, 2000, pp. 2396–2407.
6. H. Zhang, J. K. Jackson, and M. Chiao, "Microfabricated drug delivery devices: design, fabrication, and applications," *Advanced Functional Materials*, vol. 27, no. 45, 2017, pp. 1703606.

7. K. Ramesh, S. Gupta, S. Ahmed, and V. Kakkar, "A comprehensive study on design trends and future scope of implantable drug delivery systems," *International Journal of Bio-Science and Bio-Technology*, vol. 8, no. 6, 2016, pp. 11–20.
8. K. Y. Zhu, H. Zheng, and D. G. Zhang, "A computerized drug delivery control system for regulation of blood pressure," *International Journal of Intelligent Computing in Medical Sciences & Image Processing*, vol. 2, no. 1, 2008, pp. 1–13.
9. Y. Chahibi, M. Pierobon, S. O. Song, and I. F. Akyildiz, "A molecular communication system model for particulate drug delivery systems," *IEEE Transactions on Biomedical Engineering*, vol. 60, no. 12, 2013, pp. 3468–3483.
10. D. Liu, H. Zhang, F. Fontana, J. T. Hirvonen, and H. A. Santos, "Microfluidic-assisted fabrication of carriers for controlled drug delivery," *Lab on a Chip*, vol. 17, no. 11, 2017, pp. 1856–1883.
11. T. Nisisako, "Recent advances in microfluidic production of Janus droplets and particles," *Current Opinion in Colloid & Interface Science*, vol. 25, 2016, pp. 1–12.
12. J. H. Prescott, S. Lipka, S. Baldwin, N. F. Sheppard Jr, J. M. Maloney, J. Coppeta, and J. T. Santini Jr, "Chronic, programmed polypeptide delivery from an implanted, multireservoir microchip device," *Nature Biotechnology*, vol. 24, no. 4, 2006, pp. 437–438.
13. T. Hastie, J. Friedman, and R. Tibshirani, "Kernel methods," in *The Elements of Statistical Learning: Data Mining, Inference, and Prediction*, T. Hastie, J. Friedman, and R. Tibshirani, Eds. New York: Springer, 2001, pp. 165–192.
14. P. Grant, "A new approach to diabetic control: fuzzy logic and insulin pump technology," *Medical Engineering & Physics*, vol. 29, no. 7, 2007, pp. 824–827.
15. S. Nihar, P. Nishith, and K. R. Patel, "A sequential review on intelligent drug delivery system," *Journal of Pharmaceutical Science and Bioscientific Research*, vol. 3, no. 5, 2013, pp. 158–162.
16. E. Murtoniemi, P. Merkku, P. Kinnunen, K. Leiviskä, and J. Yliruusi, "Effect of neural network topology and training end point in modelling the fluidized bed granulation process," *International Journal of Pharmaceutics*, vol. 110, no. 2, 1994, pp. 101–108.
17. A. S. Achanta, J. G. Kowalski, and C. T. Rhodes, "Artificial neural networks: implications for pharmaceutical sciences," *Drug Development and Industrial Pharmacy*, vol. 21, no. 1, 1995, pp. 119–155.
18. A. Heller, "Integrated medical feedback systems for drug delivery," *AIChE Journal*, vol. 51, no. 4, 2005, pp. 1054–1066.
19. A. Sherriff, J. Ott, and ALSPAC Study Team, "Artificial neural networks as statistical tools in epidemiological studies: analysis of risk factors for early infant wheeze," *Paediatric and Perinatal Epidemiology*, vol. 18, no. 6, 2004, pp. 456–463.
20. D. S. Char, N. H. Shah, and D. Magnus, "Implementing machine learning in health care—addressing ethical challenges," *The New England Journal of Medicine*, vol. 378, no. 11, 2018, pp. 981.RetryClaude can make mistakes. Please double-check responses. 3.7 Sonnet
21. J. Bali, R. Garg, and R. T. Bali, "Artificial intelligence (AI) in healthcare and biomedical research: Why a strong computational/AI bioethics framework is required?" *Indian Journal of Ophthalmology*, vol. 67, no. 1, 2019, pp. 3–6.

22. N. T. Wilson, "No longer science fiction, AI and robotics are transforming healthcare." *PWC*, 2017. Accessed October 31, 2021.
23. G. V. K. S. Abhinav and S. N. Subrahmanyam, "Artificial intelligence in healthcare." *Journal of Drug Delivery and Therapeutics*, vol. 9, no. 5s, 2019, pp. 164–166.
24. R. Gupta, D. Srivastava, M. Sahu, S. Tiwari, R. K. Ambasta, and P. Kumar, "Artificial intelligence to deep learning: machine intelligence approach for drug discovery." *Molecular Diversity*, vol. 25, 2021, pp. 1315–1360.
25. A. I. Tekkeşin, "Artificial intelligence in healthcare: past, present and future," Anatolian Journal of Cardiology, vol. 22(Suppl 2), pp. 8–9.
26. N. O. M. Sadiku, O. I. Fagbohungbe, and S. M. Musa, "Artificial intelligence in healthcare: an overview," *International Journal of Engineering Research and Advanced Technology*, vol. 6, no. 12, 2020, pp. 38–45.
27. T. Davenport and R. Kalakota, "The potential for artificial intelligence in healthcare," *Future Healthcare Journal*, vol. 6, no. 2, 2019, p. 94.
28. S. Reddy, "Use of artificial intelligence in healthcare delivery," *eHealth-Making Health Care Smarter*, IntechOpen, 2018.
29. Y. Freund and R. E. Schapire, "Experiments with a new boosting algorithm," *ICML*, vol. 96, 1996, pp. 148–156.
30. J. H. Friedman, "Stochastic gradient boosting," *Computational Statistics & Data Analysis*, vol. 38, no. 4, 2002, pp. 367–378.
31. T. Chen and C. Guestrin, "Xgboost: A scalable tree boosting system," Proceedings of the 22nd ACM SIGKDD International Conference on Knowledge Discovery and Data Mining, 2016, pp. 785–794.
32. L. Prokhorenkova, G. Gusev, A. Vorobev, A. V. Dorogush, and A. Gulin, "CatBoost: unbiased boosting with categorical features," *Advances in Neural Information Processing Systems*, vol. 31, 2018.
33. A. J. Myles, R. N. Feudale, Y. Liu, N. A. Woody, and S. D. Brown, "An introduction to decision tree modeling," *Journal of Chemometrics: A Journal of the Chemometrics Society*, vol. 18, no. 6, 2004, pp. 275–285.
34. J. R. Quinlan, "Induction of decision trees," *Machine Learning*, vol. 1, 1986, pp. 81–106.
35. J. R. Quinlan, "C4.5: programs for machine learning," in *Machine Learning*, Elsevier, 2014.
36. D. Steinberg, "CART: classification and regression trees," *The Top Ten Algorithms in Data Mining*, 2009, pp. 193–216.
37. L. Breiman, "Random forests," *Machine Learning*, vol. 45, no. 1, 2001, pp. 5–32.
38. R. Rahman, K. Matlock, S. Ghosh, and R. Pal, "Heterogeneity aware random forest for drug sensitivity prediction," *Scientific Reports*, vol. 7, no. 1, 2017, pp. 11347.
39. S. Huang, N. Cai, P. P. Pacheco, S. Narrandes, Y. Wang, and W. Xu, "Applications of support vector machine (SVM) learning in cancer genomics," *Cancer Genomics & Proteomics*, vol. 15, no. 1, 2018, pp. 41–51.
40. T. Cover and P. Hart, "Nearest neighbor pattern classification," *IEEE Transactions on Information Theory*, vol. 13, no. 1, 1967, pp. 21–27.
41. L. Liu, X. Hu, Z. Feng, X. Zhang, S. Wang, S. Xu, and K. Sun, "Prediction of acid radical ion binding residues by K-nearest neighbors classifier," *BMC Molecular and Cell Biology*, vol. 20, 2019, pp. 1–10.

42. M. Pavlou, G. Ambler, S. Seaman, M. De Iorio, and R. Z. Omar, "Review and evaluation of penalised regression methods for risk prediction in low-dimensional data with few events," *Statistics in Medicine*, vol. 35, no. 7, 2016, pp. 1159–1177.
43. Y. Choi and Y. Boo, "Comparing logistic regression models with alternative machine learning methods to predict the risk of drug intoxication mortality," *International Journal of Environmental Research and Public Health*, vol. 17, no. 3, 2020, pp. 897.
44. R. K. Elswick Jr, P. F. Schwartz, and J. A. Welsh, "Interpretation of the odds ratio from logistic regression after a transformation of the covariate vector," *Statistics in Medicine*, vol. 16, no. 15, 1997, pp. 1695–1703.
45. J. Ren, Z. Ning, C. S. Kirkness, C. V. Asche, and H. Wang, "Risk of using logistic regression to illustrate exposure-response relationship of infectious diseases," *BMC Infectious Diseases*, vol. 14, 2014, pp. 1–8.
46. K. Hornik, M. Stinchcombe, and H. White, "Multilayer feedforward networks are universal approximators," *Neural Networks*, vol. 2, no. 5, 1989, pp. 359–366.
47. Y. LeCun, Y. Bengio, and G. Hinton, "Deep learning," *Nature*, vol. 521, no. 7553, 2015, pp. 436–444.
48. A. Drouin, S. Giguère, M. Déraspe, M. Marchand, M. Tyers, V. G. Loo, and J. Corbeil, "Predictive computational phenotyping and biomarker discovery using reference-free genome comparisons," *BMC Genomics*, vol. 17, 2016, pp. 1–15.
49. P. Nowak-Sliwinska, A. Weiss, X. Ding, P. J. Dyson, H. Van Den Bergh, A. W. Griffioen, and C. M. Ho, "Optimization of drug combinations using feedback system control," *Nature Protocols*, vol. 11, no. 2, 2016, pp. 302–315.
50. X. Ding, Z. Njus, T. Kong, W. Su, C. M. Ho, and S. Pandey, "Effective drug combination for Caenorhabditis elegans nematodes discovered by output-driven feedback system control technique," *Science Advances*, vol. 3, no. 10, 2017, pp. 1254.
51. N. Malagutti, A. Dehghani, and R. A. Kennedy, "Robust control design for automatic regulation of blood pressure," *IET Control Theory & Applications*, vol. 7, no. 3, 2013, pp. 387–396.
52. H. R. Warner, A. F. Toronto, L. G. Veasey, and R. Stephenson, "A mathematical approach to medical diagnosis: application to congenital heart disease," *JAMA*, vol. 177, no. 3, 1961, pp. 177–183.
53. B. Ehsani-Moghaddam, J. A. Queenan, J. MacKenzie, and R. V. Birtwhistle, "Mucopolysaccharidosis type II detection by Naïve Bayes Classifier: An example of patient classification for a rare disease using electronic medical records from the Canadian Primary Care Sentinel Surveillance Network," *PLoS One*, vol. 13, no. 12, 2018, pp. 18.
54. P. N. Bennet, "Assessing the calibration of Naive Bayes' posterior estimates," *School of Computer Science*, Carnegie Mellon University, 2000, pp. 0010.
55. G. M. Sacha and P. Varona, "Artificial intelligence in nanotechnology," *Nanotechnology*, vol. 24, no. 45, 2013, pp. 452002.
56. D. Q. Ly, L. Paramonov, C. Davidson, J. Ramsden, H. Wright, and N. Holliman, "Nanotechnology perception," *Nanotechnology Perceptions*, vol. 7, 2011, pp. 199–217.

57. J. M. Wing, "Computational thinking and thinking about computing," *Philosophical Transactions of the Royal Society A: Mathematical, Physical and Engineering Sciences*, vol. 366, no. 1881, 2008, pp. 3717–3725.
58. A. Aliper, S. Plis, A. Artemov, A. Ulloa, P. Mamoshina, and A. Zhavoronkov, "Deep learning applications for predicting pharmacological properties of drugs and drug repurposing using transcriptomic data," *Molecular Pharmaceutics*, vol. 13, no. 7, 2016, pp. 2524–2530.
59. N. Fleming, "Computer-calculated compounds," *Nature*, vol. 557, no. 7707, 2018, pp. S55–S57.
60. T. Van Laarhoven and E. Marchiori, "Predicting drug-target interactions for new drug compounds using a weighted nearest neighbor profile," *PLoS One*, vol. 8, no. 6, 2013, pp. e66952.
61. Z. Xia, L. Y. Wu, X. Zhou, and S. T. Wong, "Semi-supervised drug-protein interaction prediction from heterogeneous biological spaces," *BMC Systems Biology*, vol. 4, BioMed Central, 2010, pp. 1–16.
62. T. Van Laarhoven, S. B. Nabuurs, and E. Marchiori, "Gaussian interaction profile kernels for predicting drug–target interaction," *Bioinformatics*, vol. 27, no. 21, 2011, pp. 3036–3043.
63. P. Valeh-e-Sheyda, F. Yaripour, G. Moradi, and M. Saber, "Application of artificial neural networks for estimation of the reaction rate in methanol dehydration," *Industrial & Engineering Chemistry Research*, vol. 49, no. 10, 2010, pp. 4620–4626.
64. T. Fox and J. M. Kriegl, "Machine learning techniques for in silico modeling of drug metabolism," *Current Topics in Medicinal Chemistry*, vol. 6, no. 15, 2006, pp. 1579–1591.
65. G. Von Maltzahn, J. H. Park, K. Y. Lin, N. Singh, C. Schwöppe, R. Mesters, and S. N. Bhatia, "Nanoparticles that communicate in vivo to amplify tumour targeting," *Nature Materials*, vol. 10, no. 7, 2011, pp. 545–552.
66. X. Liu, P. Lin, I. Perrett, J. Lin, Y. P. Liao, C. H. Chang, and H. Meng, "Tumor-penetrating peptide enhances transcytosis of silicasome-based chemotherapy for pancreatic cancer," *The Journal of Clinical Investigation*, vol. 127, no. 5, 2017, pp. 2007–2018.
67. X. Xu, K. Xie, X. Q. Zhang, E. M. Pridgen, G. Y. Park, D. S. Cui, and O. C. Farokhzad, "Enhancing tumor cell response to chemotherapy through nanoparticle-mediated codelivery of siRNA and cisplatin prodrug," *Proceedings of the National Academy of Sciences*, vol. 110, no. 46, 2013, pp. 18638–18643.
68. W. Fan, B. Shen, W. Bu, F. Chen, K. Zhao, S. Zhang, and J. Shi, "Rattle-structured multifunctional nanotheranostics for synergetic chemo-/radiotherapy and simultaneous magnetic/luminescent dual-mode imaging," *Journal of the American Chemical Society*, vol. 135, no. 17, 2013, pp. 6494–6503.
69. H. Wang, D. K. Lee, K. Y. Chen, J. Y. Chen, K. Zhang, A. Silva, and D. Ho, "Mechanism-independent optimization of combinatorial nanodiamond and unmodified drug delivery using a phenotypically driven platform technology," *ACS Nano*, vol. 9, no. 3, 2015, pp. 3332–3344.
70. P. Hassanzadeh, F. Atyabi, and R. Dinarvand, "The significance of artificial intelligence in drug delivery system design," *Advanced Drug Delivery Reviews*, vol. 151, 2019, pp. 169–190.

71. M. Luo, Y. Feng, T. Wang, and J. Guan, "Micro-/nanorobots at work in active drug delivery," *Advanced Functional Materials*, vol. 28, no. 25, 2018, pp. 1706100.
72. J. Fu and H. Yan, "Controlled drug release by a nanorobot," *Nature Biotechnology*, vol. 30, no. 5, 2012, pp. 407–408.
73. X. Jin, D. D. Zhu, B. Z. Chen, M. Ashfaq, and X. D. Guo, "Insulin delivery systems combined with microneedle technology," *Advanced Drug Delivery Reviews*, vol. 127, 2018, pp. 119–137.
74. T. Sekigami, S. Shimoda, K. Nishida, Y. Matsuo, S. Ichimori, K. Ichinose, and E. Araki, "Comparison between closed-loop portal and peripheral venous insulin delivery systems for an artificial endocrine pancreas," *Journal of Artificial Organs*, vol. 7, 2004, pp. 91–100.
75. R. Sharma, D. Singh, P. Gaur, and D. Joshi, "Intelligent automated drug administration and therapy: future of healthcare," *Drug Delivery and Translational Research*, 2021, pp. 1–25.
76. G. I. Voss, "Closed loop drug delivery: an industry perspective," Proceedings of the Twelfth Annual International Conference of the IEEE Engineering in Medicine and Biology Society, IEEE, 1990, pp. 940–940.
77. B. Kovatchev, "Automated closed-loop control of diabetes: the artificial pancreas," *Bioelectronic Medicine*, vol. 4, no. 1, 2018, p. 14.
78. P. Sundaravadivel, E. Kougianos, S. P. Mohanty, and M. K. Ganapathiraju, "Everything you wanted to know about smart health care: Evaluating the different technologies and components of the internet of things for better health," *IEEE Consumer Electronics Magazine*, vol. 7, no. 1, 2017, pp. 18–28.
79. I. B. Abbes, P. Y. Richard, M. A. Lefebvre, I. Guilhem, and J. Y. Poirier, "A closed-loop artificial pancreas using a proportional integral derivative with double phase lead controller based on a new nonlinear model of glucose metabolism," *Journal of Diabetes Science and Technology*, vol. 7, no. 3, 2013, pp. 699–707.
80. F. Chee, A. V. Savkin, T. L. Fernando, and S. Nahavandi, "Optimal H/sup/ spl infin//insulin injection control for blood glucose regulation in diabetic patients," *IEEE Transactions on Biomedical Engineering*, vol. 52, no. 10, 2005, pp. 1625–1631.
81. R. Dudde and T. Vering, "Advanced insulin infusion using a control loop (ADICOL) concept and realization of a control-loop application for the automated delivery of insulin," 4th International IEEE EMBS Special Topic Conference on Information Technology Applications in Biomedicine, IEEE, 2003, pp. 280–282.
82. A. Abu-Rmileh, W. Garcia-Gabin, and D. Zambrano, "Internal model sliding mode control approach for glucose regulation in type 1 diabetes," *Biomedical Signal Processing and Control*, vol. 5, no. 2, 2010, pp. 94–102.
83. D. U. Campos-Delgado, M. Hernández-Ordoñez, R. Femat, and A. Gordillo-Moscoso, "Fuzzy-based controller for glucose regulation in type-1 diabetic patients by subcutaneous route," in *IEEE Transactions on Biomedical Engineering*, vol. 53, no. 11, 2006, pp. 2201–2210.
84. B. S. Leon, A. Y. Alanis, E. N. Sanchez, F. Ornelas-Tellez, and E. Ruiz-Velazquez, "Inverse optimal neural control of blood glucose level for type 1 diabetes mellitus patients," *Journal of the Franklin Institute*, vol. 349, no. 5, 2012, pp. 1851–1870.

85. P. Kaveh and Y. B. Shtessel, "Blood glucose regulation in diabetics using sliding mode control techniques," Proceeding of the Thirty-Eighth Southeastern Symposium on System Theory, IEEE, 2006, pp. 171–175.
86. S. Yasini, A. Karimpour, M. B. Naghibi-Sistani, and S. Ghareh, "An automatic insulin infusion system based on H-infinity control technique," Cairo International Biomedical Engineering Conference, IEEE, 2008, pp. 1–5.
87. S. Zavitsanou, A. Mantalaris, M. C. Georgiadis, and E. N. Pistikopoulos, "In silico closed-loop control validation studies for optimal insulin delivery in type 1 diabetes," *IEEE Transactions on Biomedical Engineering*, vol. 62, no. 10, 2015, pp. 2369–2378.
88. D. Shi, E. Dassau, and F. J. Doyle, "Adaptive zone model predictive control of artificial pancreas based on glucose-and velocity-dependent control penalties," *IEEE Transactions on Biomedical Engineering*, vol. 66, no. 4, 2018, pp. 1045–1054.
89. H. Thabit and R. Hovorka, "Closed-loop insulin delivery in type 1 diabetes," *Endocrinology and Metabolism Clinics*, vol. 41, no. 1, 2012, pp. 105–117.
90. K. Scholten and E. Meng, "A review of implantable biosensors for closed-loop glucose control and other drug delivery applications," *International Journal of Pharmaceutics*, vol. 544, no. 2, 2018, pp. 319–334.
91. G. A. Giridharan and M. Skliar, "Nonlinear controller for ventricular assist devices," *Artificial Organs*, vol. 26, no. 11, 2002, pp. 980–984.
92. M. I. Elnaggar, A. S. Ashour, Y. Guo, H. A. El-Khobby, and M. M. Abd Elnaby, "An optimized Mamdani FPD controller design of cardiac pacemaker," *Health Information Science and Systems*, vol. 7, 2019, pp. 1–18.
93. C. P. Valcke and H. J. Chizeck, "Closed-loop drug infusion for control of heart-rate trajectory in pharmacological stress tests," *IEEE Transactions on Biomedical Engineering*, vol. 44, no. 3, 1997, pp. 185–195.
94. D. M. Cosgrove III, J. H. Petre, J. L. Waller, J. V. Roth, C. Shepherd, and L. H. Cohn, "Automated control of postoperative hypertension: a prospective, randomized multicenter study," *The Annals of Thoracic Surgery*, vol. 47, no. 5, 1989, pp. 678–683.
95. C. T. Chen, W. L. Lin, T. S. Kuo, and C. Y. Wang, "Adaptive control of arterial blood pressure with a learning controller based on multilayer neural networks," *IEEE Transactions on Biomedical Engineering*, vol. 44, no. 7, 1997, pp. 601–609.RetryClaude can make mistakes. Please double-check responses. 3.7 Sonnet
96. H. Ying, M. McEachern, D. W. Eddleman, and L. C. Sheppard, "Fuzzy control of mean arterial pressure in postsurgical patients with sodium nitroprusside infusion," *IEEE Transactions on Biomedical Engineering*, vol. 39, no. 10, 1992, pp. 1060–1070.
97. C. W. Frei, M. Derighetti, M. Morari, A. H. Glattfelder, and A. M. Zbinden, "Improving regulation of mean arterial blood pressure during anesthesia through estimates of surgery effects," *IEEE Transactions on Biomedical Engineering*, vol. 47, no. 11, 2000, pp. 1456–1464.
98. S. Sondhi and Y. V. Hote, "Fractional-order PI controller with specific gain–phase margin for MABP control," *IETE Journal of Research*, vol. 61, no. 2, 2015, pp. 142–153.

99. J. M. Arnsparger, B. C. Mcinnis, J. R. Glover, and N. A. Normann, "Adaptive control of blood pressure," *IEEE Transactions on Biomedical Engineering*, no. 3, 1983, pp. 168–176.
100. G. A. Pajunen, M. Steinmetz, and R. Shankar, "Model reference adaptive control with constraints for postoperative blood pressure management," *IEEE Transactions on Biomedical Engineering*, vol. 37, no. 7, 1990, pp. 679–687.
101. R. Padmanabhan, N. Meskin, and W. M. Haddad, "Closed-loop control of anesthesia and mean arterial pressure using reinforcement learning," *Biomedical Signal Processing and Control*, vol. 22, 2015, pp. 54–64.
102. K. E. Kwok, S. L. Shah, B. A. Finegan, and G. K. Kwong, "An observational trial of a computerized drug delivery system on two patients," *IEEE Transactions on Control Systems Technology*, vol. 5, no. 4, 1997, pp. 385–393.
103. M. M. Polycarpou and J. Y. Conway, "Indirect adaptive nonlinear control of drug delivery systems," *IEEE Transactions on Automatic Control*, vol. 43, no. 6, 1998, pp. 849–856.
104. C. Treesatayapun, "Minimized sodium nitroprusside for mean arterial pressure regulation based on fuzzy rules emulated networks," *Applied Mathematical Modelling*, vol. 34, no. 5, 2010, pp. 1292–1310.
105. Y. Gao and M. J. Er, "An intelligent adaptive control scheme for postsurgical blood pressure regulation," *IEEE Transactions on Neural Networks*, vol. 16, no. 2, 2005, pp. 475–483.
106. F. J. Doyle III, B. W. Bequette, R. Middleton, B. Ogunnaike, B. Paden, R. S. Parker, and M. Vidyasagar, "Control in biological systems," *The Impact of Control Technology*, 2011.
107. J. R. Boston, M. A. Simaan, J. F. Antaki, and Y. C. Yu, "Control issues in rotary heart assist devices," Proceedings of the 2000 American Control Conference, IEEE, vol. 5, 2000, pp. 3473–3477.
108. X. Guo, Z. Luo, H. Cui, J. Wang, and Q. Jiang, "A novel and reproducible release mechanism for a drug-delivery system in the gastrointestinal tract," *Biomedical Microdevices*, vol. 21, 2019, pp. 1–9.
109. S. P. Woods and T. G. Constandinou, "Wireless capsule endoscope for targeted drug delivery: mechanics and design considerations," *IEEE Transactions on Biomedical Engineering*, vol. 60, no. 4, 2012, pp. 945–953.
110. G. D. Meron, "The development of the swallowable video capsule (M2A)," *Gastrointestinal Endoscopy*, vol. 52, no. 6, 2000, pp. 817–819.
111. P. Swain and A. Fritscher-Ravens, "Role of video endoscopy in managing small bowel disease," *Gut*, vol. 53, no. 12, 2004, pp. 1866–1875.
112. G. Tortora, B. Orsini, P. Pecile, A. Menciassi, F. Fusi, and G. Romano, "An ingestible capsule for the photodynamic therapy of helicobacter pylori infection," *IEEE/ASME Transactions on Mechatronics*, vol. 21, no. 4, 2016, pp. 1935–1942.
113. B. Li and M. Q. H. Meng, "Tumor recognition in wireless capsule endoscopy images using textural features and SVM-based feature selection," *IEEE Transactions on Information Technology in Biomedicine*, vol. 16, no. 3, 2012, pp. 323–329.
114. D. Becker, J. Zhang, T. Heimbach, R. C. Penland, C. Wanke, J. Shimizu, and K. Kulmatycki, "Novel orally swallowable IntelliCap® device to quantify regional drug absorption in human GI tract using diltiazem as model drug," *AAPS PharmSciTech*, vol. 15, 2014, pp. 1490–1497.

115. V. H. Le, H. L. Rodriguez, C. Lee, G. Go, J. Zhen, H. Choi, and S. Park, "A soft-magnet-based drug-delivery module for active locomotive intestinal capsule endoscopy using an electromagnetic actuation system," *Sensors and Actuators A: Physical*, vol. 243, 2016, pp. 81–89.
116. B. H. Leung, C. C. Poon, R. Zhang, Y. Zheng, C. K. Chan, P. W. Chiu, and J. J. Sung, "A therapeutic wireless capsule for treatment of gastrointestinal haemorrhage by balloon tamponade effect," *IEEE Transactions on Biomedical Engineering*, vol. 64, no. 5, 2016, pp. 1106–1114.
117. R. Goffredo, D. Accoto, and E. Guglielmelli, "Swallowable smart pills for local drug delivery: present status and future perspectives," *Expert Review of Medical Devices*, vol. 12, no. 5, 2015, pp. 585–599.
118. J. L. Gonzalez-Guillaumin, D. C. Sadowski, K. V. Kaler, and M. P. Mintchev, "Ingestible capsule for impedance and pH monitoring in the esophagus," *IEEE Transactions on Biomedical Engineering*, vol. 54, no. 12, 2007, pp. 2231–2236.
119. H. Luo, G. Xu, C. Li, L. He, L. Luo, Z. Wang, and R. H. Xu, "Real-time artificial intelligence for detection of upper gastrointestinal cancer by endoscopy: a multicentre, case-control, diagnostic study," *The Lancet Oncology*, vol. 20, no. 12, 2019, pp. 1645–1654.
120. S. Soffer, E. Klang, O. Shimon, N. Nachmias, R. Eliakim, S. Ben-Horin, and Y. Barash, "Deep learning for wireless capsule endoscopy: a systematic review and meta-analysis," *Gastrointestinal Endoscopy*, vol. 92, no. 4, 2020, pp. 831–839.
121. P. Dua, V. Dua, and E. N. Pistikopoulos, "Optimal delivery of chemotherapeutic agents in cancer," *Computers & Chemical Engineering*, vol. 32, no. 1–2, 2008, pp. 99–107.
122. M. Sharifi and H. Moradi, "Nonlinear composite adaptive control of cancer chemotherapy with online identification of uncertain parameters," *Biomedical Signal Processing and Control*, vol. 49, 2019, pp. 360–374.
123. N. Pachauri, J. Yadav, A. Rani, and V. Singh, "Modified fractional order IMC design based drug scheduling for cancer treatment," *Computers in Biology and Medicine*, vol. 109, 2019, pp. 121–137.
124. F. S. Lobato, V. S. Machado, and V. Steffen Jr, "Determination of an optimal control strategy for drug administration in tumor treatment using multi-objective optimization differential evolution," *Computer Methods and Programs in Biomedicine*, vol. 131, 2016, pp. 51–61.
125. B. Bojkov, R. Hansel, and R. Luus, "Application of direct search optimization to optimal control problems," *Hungarian Journal of Industrial Chemistry*, vol. 21, 1993, pp. 177–177.
126. S. Algoul, M. S. Alam, M. A. Hossain, and M. A. A. Majumder, "Multi-objective optimal chemotherapy control model for cancer treatment," *Medical & Biological Engineering & Computing*, vol. 49, 2011, pp. 51–65.
127. A. H. El-Garawany, M. E. Karar, and M. A. El-Brawany, "Embedded drug delivery controller for cancer chemotherapy under treatment constrains," 2017 International Conference on Advanced Control Circuits Systems (ACCS) Systems & 2017 International Conference on New Paradigms in Electronics & Information Technology (PEIT), IEEE, 2017, pp. 264–271.
128. S. Khadraoui, F. Harrou, H. N. Nounou, M. N. Nounou, A. Datta, and S. P. Bhattacharyya, "A measurement-based control design approach for efficient cancer chemotherapy," *Information Sciences*, vol. 333, 2016, pp. 108–125.

129. H. Nasiri and A. A. Kalat, "Adaptive fuzzy back-stepping control of drug dosage regimen in cancer treatment," *Biomedical Signal Processing and Control*, vol. 42, 2018, pp. 267–276.
130. R. Padmanabhan, N. Meskin, and W. M. Haddad, "Learning-based control of cancer chemotherapy treatment," *IFAC-PapersOnLine*, vol. 50, no. 1, 2017, pp. 15127–15132.
131. P. Khalili and R. Vatankhah, "Derivation of an optimal trajectory and nonlinear adaptive controller design for drug delivery in cancerous tumor chemotherapy," *Computers in Biology and Medicine*, vol. 109, 2019, pp. 195–206.
132. B. Ramkumar and D. S. Naidu, "Closed-loop optimal control strategy for cancer chemotherapy," *ASME International Mechanical Engineering Congress and Exposition*, vol. 43033, 2007, pp. 223–231.
133. H. Mahmoodian, S. Salem, and K. Shojaei, "Adaptively adjusted footprint of uncertainty in interval type 2 fuzzy controller for cancer drug delivery," *Procedia Computer Science*, vol. 76, 2015, pp. 360–367.
134. J. A. Florian Jr, J. L. Eiseman, and R. S. Parker, "Nonlinear model predictive control for dosing daily anticancer agents using a novel saturating-rate cell-cycle model," *Computers in Biology and Medicine*, vol. 38, no. 3, 2008, pp. 339–347.
135. R. Padmanabhan, N. Meskin, and W. M. Haddad, "Reinforcement learning-based control of drug dosing for cancer chemotherapy treatment," *Mathematical Biosciences*, vol. 293, 2017, pp. 11–20.
136. P. Khalili, R. Vatankhah, and S. Taghvaei, "Optimal sliding mode control of drug delivery in cancerous tumour chemotherapy considering the obesity effects," *IET Systems Biology*, vol. 12, no. 4, 2018, pp. 185–189.
137. B. S. Dey, M. K. Bera, and B. K. Roy, "Super twisting sliding mode control of cancer chemotherapy," 2018 15th International Workshop on Variable Structure Systems (VSS), IEEE, 2018, pp. 343–348.
138. L. Kovács, A. Szeles, J. Sápi, D. A. Drexler, I. Rudas, I. Harmati, and Z. Sápi, "Model-based angiogenic inhibition of tumor growth using modern robust control method," *Computer Methods and Programs in Biomedicine*, vol. 114, no. 3, 2014, pp. e98–e110.
139. P. Vivek, P. Nikhil, R. Asha, and S. Vijander, "Optimal ISA-PID-based drug concentration control in cancer chemotherapy," Intelligent Communication, Control and Devices: Proceedings of ICICCD 2017, Springer Singapore, 2018, pp. 165–171.
140. P. L. Mage, B. S. Ferguson, D. Maliniak, K. L. Ploense, T. E. Kippin, and H. T. Soh, "Closed-loop control of circulating drug levels in live animals," *Nature Biomedical Engineering*, vol. 1, no. 5, 2017, pp. 0070.

Chapter 8

# Artificial intelligence in genomics

*Rashmi Rameshwari, Adhikarka Syama, Srinivasan Ramachandran, Devendra Kumar Verma, and Santosh Kumar*

## 8.1 INTRODUCTION

Before exploring artificial intelligence (AI) and its role in genomics, it is essential to understand a few terminologies for better clarity. The terms "artificial intelligence" and "machine learning" (ML) are often used interchangeably. There exists a reasonable difference between the two (https://www.coursera.org/articles/machine-learning-vs-ai).

**AI**: A field that mimics human thinking and performs tasks such as language interpretation, data analysis, and decision-making. AI serves as an umbrella that encompasses various technologies such as ML, deep learning (DL), and natural language processing (NLP). Examples include ChatGPT, Google Translate, NETFLIX, and TESLA.

**ML**: A subfield of AI that defines methods to perform specific tasks. It uses algorithms on datasets and predictive models to perform a task. The models are created by training algorithms such as supervised, unsupervised, semi-supervised, and reinforcement learning (https://www.coursera.org/articles/machine-learning-models). Examples of ML include face recognition, email spam filtering, website product recommendations, social media optimization, etc.

**DL**: A subfield of ML that uses artificial neural networks to mimic the human brain to perform a task without human intervention. Examples are speech recognition, and pattern recognition in images and text.

**NLP**: A subfield of computer science, AI, ML, and linguistics. It focuses on creating a platform for interpreting human communication. Examples include Chatbots for customer service with spoken commands, voice-operated GPS, digital assistants on smartphones, etc.

**Robotics**: A field using AI, computer science, and electrical engineering to create robots capable of learning and performing complex tasks.


DOI: 10.1201/9781003741770-8

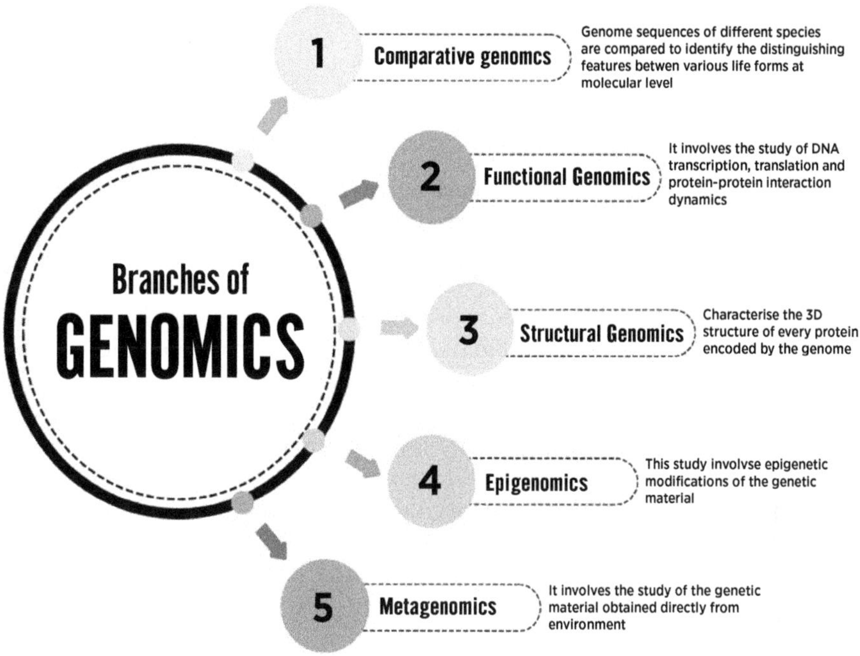


*Figure 8.1* Different branches of genomics

**Genomics:** An interdisciplinary field involving the study of structure, function, evolution, mapping, and editing at the genome level. It has several sub-branches, as shown in Figure 8.1. The data collected through genomic studies find applications in genomic medicine, synthetic biology, evolutionary genomics, population, and conservation genomics.

## 8.2 WHAT IS AI?

Artificial intelligence (AI) is a technology that enables computers and machines to perform complex tasks that otherwise require human intervention, including self-awareness, logic, and learning from experience. Alan Turing imagined a human-like machine that could work according to the coded program and beyond. He even developed a machine called Bombe (meaning to decode). This machine was deployed during the Second World War to crack German codes on military operations. The concept of "thinking machines" was discussed at the Dartmouth conference, arousing their peers' excitement. In 1956, John McCarthy coined the term "artificial intelligence." Over the next two decades, there has been a huge development in AI [1–3].

## 8.3 BIOLOGY-INSPIRED AI

Let us now peek into the relationship between AI and biology. In 1943, Warren McCulloh and Walter Pitts published their research paper titled "A Logical Calculus of the Ideas Immanent in Nervous Activity" in the *Bulletin of Mathematical Biophysics* [4]. In this article, the authors applied a mathematical model for the functioning of a single neuron, thereby establishing a connection between biological processes and computation. Later, in the 1950s, Frank Rosenblatt asked himself a question, "What are the minimum number of things that a brain need to have physically to perform a task?" Thus, he developed a single-layer neural network algorithm called Perceptron, which predicted the directions (right or left) or objects (dog or cat) [5]. The accuracy of this system could be improved by several iterations. Later, two independent works by Hubel and Wiesel [6] and Fukushima [7] built models on the human visual cortex and pattern recognition. Thus, it is clear that the biological process did inspire the generation of AI [8]. However, the mimicking biological process has not been limited to the neurological system but has extended to the human immune system and other species like plants and microbes. However, in this chapter, we will focus on the development of AI in genomics and its applications.

## 8.4 WHY USE AI, ML, AND ANN IN GENOMICS?

Biology is incredibly complex. This is in term of numer of variations, no of component with respect to time and space. Additionally, technologies such as PCR, Sanger sequencing, next-generation sequencing (NGS), and other omics technology platforms have enormously increased the volume of data.

The human genome project, which was completed in 2003, sequenced 3 billion DNA letters in the human genome with an accuracy of 99.99%. Following this, NIH estimates that the genomic research will generate 2 to 40 exabytes of data within the next decade (https://www.genome.gov/). The upcoming technologies are likely to increase the complexity of the data.

Hence, to derive meaningful genomics insights from the data, a robust technology has to be developed. AI is one such technology that comes to our rescue. This helps us *automate* certain processes to *obtain reproducible results* and *save time*. It enables us to *dive deep into data* that would otherwise not be possible with human eyes, thereby *decreasing errors*. Conversely, aggressive development of AI tools to better meet the data analysis requirements is being undertaken.

## 8.5 CHRONOLOGICAL ORDER OF AI APPLICATION IN THE AREA OF GENOMICS

The digitalizing of life sciences started around 1949 [9]. The first laboratory-installed computer at the Massachusetts Institute was built in 1962, which transformed biological research. An American molecular biologist and Nobel laureate, Joshua Lederberg, collaborated with NASA to interpret data to find life on Mars. In this context, he realized that mass spectrometry could be a powerful technology to identify organic molecules. However, the materials of Mars could not be compared with those on Earth. So the necessity arose to develop a mechanism to identify new compounds. This led to the development of an early application of AI called DENDRAL in 1964. This program would generate possible chemical structures from mass spectrometric data [10]. In the 1970s, researchers at Stanford University attempted to diagnose patients based on their symptoms and medical test reports. Edward H. Shortliffe came up with a rule-based expert system called MYCIN, which used AI and a model of interaction between physicians and human consultants [11]. MYCIN's area of expertise was in the selection of antimicrobial therapy for patients with severe infections. Another study, conducted in 1982 by Stormo et al., used an AI tool called Perceptron to identify translation initiation sites of *Escherichia coli* from a library of 78,612 linear mRNA nucleotides residing on 124 genes [12].

Later with the discovery of DNA and first-generation sequencing technologies such as Sanger and Maxam–Gilbert sequencing, AI applications had been more focused on developing algorithms for sequence analysis and identifying genes, gene prediction, and motif discovery. The genome sequence of *Saccharomyces cerevisiae* in 1996 paved the way to explore the relationship between genes and their products. Techniques such as hidden Markov models (HMMs) were used in biological sequence analysis by Churchill to study the structure of small complete genomes such as mitochondrial DNA, bacteriophage lambda, Simian Virus (SV 40), and human genome segments such as human α-globin region [13]. Tools like Basic Local Alignment Search Tool (BLAST), developed in the early 1990s, used AI algorithms to search for similar sequences in large databases, facilitating the comparison of genetic sequences. By 2002, second-generation sequencing technologies emerged with the development of 454 GS20 sequencers. In 2011, third-generation sequencing technologies emerged with Oxford's single-molecule sequencing technology [14]. These technologies deploy changes in electric signals and translocation times to identify nitrogenous bases. Hence, there is a chance of generating noise data along with data of relevance. At this point, ML tools can be utilized to identify accurate nucleotide signals from noise. Secondly, it resolves signal overlap between current nucleotides through classification tools. Thirdly, ML tools can identify current signals from complex data with a high magnitude of noise and recognize the genetic code [15]. ML techniques such as vector machines, random forest, and deep learning algorithms are used for variant analysis, identification of disease-associated genes/variants, drug discovery, and clinical research, thereby aiding personalized medicine. The sequencing technologies have necessitated the use of AI applications for the identification of promoters, enhancers, and splice sites; annotation; cell type prediction; 3D genome folding prediction; tumor classification; RNA transcript classification; alternative splicing pattern detection; and the identification of protein structures, motifs, and sequences.

In late 2014, deep learning for a genomics model called "Chromputer" came into existence. It used convolutional neural networks (CNNs) to predict histone modifications and chromatin states from 2D DNA accessibility data. Shortly thereafter, the DeepBind and DeepSEA models were published. DeepBind [16] is a fully automatic stand-alone software for the prediction of sequence specificities of DNA- and RNA-binding proteins. DeepSEA (deep learning-based sequence analyzer) [17] predicts chromatin effects of sequence alterations at a single-nucleotide resolution by learning regulatory sequences from large-scale chromatin-profiling data. With the flooding of sequence data, databases such as ENTREZ, OMIM, GenBank, etc. evolved to store and retrieve the data effectively. Hence the tools to mine the relationship between genes, sequences, and biomedical literature started to emerge. Biological Natural Language Processing (BioNLP) creates tools and methods for the analysis of sequence and textual information. It assists in extracting latent information from biomedical literature [18] and enables the making of evidence-based decisions. It enables the identification of relevant studies, extraction of key findings, and synthesis of information for a deeper understanding of genomics.

## 8.6 CURRENT APPLICATIONS OF AI IN GENOMICS

Having seen the progress of AI tools in genomics, let us now understand how AI tools have facilitated progress in various branches of genomics.

### 8.6.1 Comparative genomics

Comparative genomics is a study that aligns and analyzes genes and genomes of extinct and/or extant species that are possibly related to varying degrees of evolutionary divergence from a common ancestor. Katsura et al. [19] studied a unique frog named *Glandirana rugosa* (Japanese wrinkled frog). This frog is unique as it has both XX-XY and ZZ-ZW sex chromosomes, indicating the possibility of system alteration. To understand the mechanism of sex turnover, the genome sequences of various frogs were compared using an unsupervised AI tool called BLSOM. This tool is effective when no prior models or knowledge is available and proved useful in identifying intraspecies differences [19].

More recently, Gao et al. developed a PrimateAI-3D, a deep-learning model trained on millions of benign primate variants from 233 primate species. Primates are evolutionarily closer to humans. Hence this algorithm identifies missense variants that are pathogenic to humans. It identifies genes that display protective/disease risk. These regions thus could be possible drug targets. Jia et al. [20] designed a panel of six genes and two single-nucleotide polymorphisms (SNPs) to distinguish between five nontuberculous mycobacteria species by combining comparative genomics and a machine learning approach. Currently, identifying these species through routine diagnosis remains a challenge. To address this, this group compared the complete genomes of 123 nontuberculosis mycobacteria and searched for specific genes/SNPs of the 5 mycobacteria under consideration using ML tools such as random forest. This model assisted in identifying combinations of genes/SNPs for discriminating species of interest. Building phylogenetic trees is very crucial in understanding the relationship between various species. Machine learning approaches such as random forest regression have been employed to guide phylogenetic tree constructions, especially when larger genomic data of multiple species are taken into consideration [21].

### 8.6.2 Functional genomics

Functional genomics deals with genome-wide scale and its relationships among biological systems such as genes, transcripts, proteins, and metabolites. It also deals with working together with all these biomolecules. Functional genomics came into existence after the first genome sequencing project. The purpose was to annotate functionally relevant features present in the sequence, such as protein coding genes, non-coding genes, and DNA regulatory regions. Over the last decade, AI has greatly enabled functional genomics, especially in "omics"-driven approaches for finding information present in sequences. It has enabled the prediction of DNA regulatory regions, the identification of associations between genotypes and phenotypes, biomarker discovery, and improved diagnosis of various diseases.

Deep learning (DL) techniques have increasingly been used in functional genomics since the second decade of the 2000s. The emergence of CRISPR-Cas9 technology for genome editing has also been accompanied by AI-driven tools for designing and optimizing genetic modifications based on personal genetic profiles. The AI models are able to predict the editing outcomes such as on-target, off-target editing. AI models and tools increase the precision, efficiency, and cost-effectiveness of editing technologies. Converting individual nucleotides in a genome without breaking the double strand [22], prime editing [23], and editing modifiers such as methylation patterns and histone modification that impact the gene function without altering gene sequence [24] are some of the advancements in gene editing technologies empowered by AI.

### 8.6.3 Structural genomics

Google-owned company DeepMind developed AI-based protein-folding prediction models called AlphaFold2, which could predict and classify deaminase proteins based on structural similarities [25]. They successfully identified two deaminase proteins, Sdd6 and Sdd7, in soybean, thus opening doors for therapeutic applications in crop genomics. The creation of edited Sdd7 transgenic plants conferred resistance to the herbicide carfentrazone-ethyl, and these plants did not show wilting [25]. AlphaFold2 can predict the structure of single proteins in minutes, down to atomic-level accuracy. This was later extended to predict the structure of protein complexes. This was a breakthrough technology that has revolutionized the field of structural genomics.

Further building on these ideas, this model was combined with trained protein language models. These language models learn the sequence information of the proteins, negating the requirement of multiple sequence alignment tools, thus enabling understanding of the structure of proteins as well as their interactions [26]. IgFold is one such example of such deep learning protein language models. It has been demonstrated that the efficacy of this model by predicting structures of 1.4 million paired antibody sequences, providing structural insights into more than 500-fold antibodies than those with experimentally determined structures [27]. A similar software, RoseTTAFold, used deep learning neural networks to compute the protein structure in less than 10 min on a single gaming laptop. This software has predicted the structures of many poorly understood proteins from the human genome, such as defective proteins associated with lipid metabolism, inflammation disorders, and cancer cell growth [28].

AI models trained on sequence and structure have been used to catalog enzymes, predict enzyme evolution and mechanisms, determine selectivity and specificity of G protein-coupled receptor (GPCRs), perform functional annotation of microbial proteins to understand their microbiome–phenotype relationships, analyze protein–membrane interfaces, predict the effects of mutations and their association with various diseases, and design new functional proteins and ligands (AI and Biology workshop 12–15 March, EMBL). However, the accuracies of these predictions are limited as these tools currently do not consider ligands, covalent modifications, and other environmental factors. It is suggested that these tools are very useful in generating hypotheses, but their predictions must be validated through laboratory experiments [29]. These tools are not yet capable of predicting protein function and folding. However, the functions of unknown proteins can be inferred from their 3D structures.

## 8.7 EPIGENOMICS

Epigenomics involves the study of heritable chemical changes that regulate DNA expression such as methylation, RNA-centered mechanisms, histone modifications, and chromatin conformation. These processes are the product of lifestyle and environment [30]. Several diseases have been associated with epigenetics, such as obesity, cardiovascular disorders, neurological disorders, etc. Machine learning techniques have helped us in finding patterns in epigenetic data of several diseases, thus facilitating the understanding of disease development, diagnosis, and treatments.

These studies are already established in oncology with FDA-approved biomarkers (e.g., SEPT 9 for colorectal cancer) as well as in diagnosis, and epigenetic therapy [26, 27]. A recent review of six epigenomic studies summariz the potential of AI in the discovery of biomarkers [27].

AI and ML algorithms have successfully identified long non-coding RNAs, especially in various cancer types, and analyzed cell type-specific DNA methylation profiles, assisting in tumor classification, predicting 3D genome folding, and identifying active and repressed genome states. Recent advances in single-cell sequencing technologies concerning genomics and epigenomics open new avenues to dissect cell heterogeneity in multiple biological processes. Recent applications of these approaches to animals and plants have provided exciting insights into diverse biological questions. Many tools have been developed that provide us information on epigenetic modifications as well as on the three major groups of DNA-binding proteins like zinc finger proteins, transcription activators like effectors and nuclease-deficient Cas9 fusion. These tools have different features and have their strengths and limitations.

## 8.8 METAGENOMICS

Metagenomics is a novel approach that combines genomics, bioinformatics, and systems biology to study the genome of many organisms at a time. After the Human Microbiome project, many microbiota were evaluated and the study has helped to find many diseases and disorders in humans. Metagenomics has also played an important role in the study of plants and microbes. The large amount of data generated by this technology is studied by machine learning tools enabled by AI to make classification and clustering of samples based on their annotations and taxonomic identifications [31].

Secondly, ML algorithms have been employed to detect antibiotic resistance genes [32, 33]. Though metagenome data is generated to study various metabolic and functional diversity, dissecting to understand the mechanism from genetic/transcriptomic information is a challenge [34]. AI rescues here by providing fast, effective, and near-accurate insights into microbial datasets. Thus identification of infectious diseases in a hospital setup at a shorter time interval is very useful.

Interestingly, identification of microbial traces from crime sites has assisted in solving crime cases and thus is one unique application of forensic medicine. Microbiota of skin, oral cavity, and intestines are highly polymorphic and specific to each individual [35, 36].

## 8.9 ARTIFICIAL INTELLIGENCE AND ITS ROLE IN INFECTIOUS DISEASES, HEALTHCARE, CANCER, PHARMACOGENOMICS, AND PRECISION MEDICINE

The tasks of healthcare professionals regarding infectious diseases include surveillance, prediction of outbreaks, identifying high-risk locations, developing preventive measures against spreading, and vaccines [37]. Artificial intelligence could aid in all these areas. Lopez-Rincon et al. [37] developed a convolutional network classifier to identify SARS-CoV-2 sequences from other virus strains accurately. Notably, 553 sequences were used to train the network. Based on the sequences used by the model to identify SARS-CoV-2, primers were designed, producing sensitivity similar to other methods and a specificity of 100%. In 2022, Scientists have [38] developed a combined method of whole genome sequencing surveillance for bacterial pathogens (about 16 species in this study) and machine learning of electronic health records to identify undetected outbreaks and transmission routes. This combined method was the Enhanced Detection System for Healthcare-Associated Transmission (EDS-HAT). Whole genome sequencing surveillance enables links between unrelated individuals, pointing to an outbreak. Machine learning and infection prevention experts can offer the transmission route. These authors claim that if EDS-HAT were implemented in real time, it would result in substantial cost savings. In 2023, Feng et al. [35 –39] report that machine-readable metadata could help identify sampling structures and thereby lead to the identification of wheels and brooms with higher proportions of samples positive for *Listeria monocytogenes*. Such data standardization and digitization could summarize high-risk locations. In 2020 scientist have been [40] used a combination of machine learning, bacterial population genomics, and genome-wide association studies and identified allelic variants corresponding to abortion-causing alleles of *porA*. The AI tools support vector machines and artificial neural networks have been used to develop several virulence factors prediction algorithms for many pathogens, including bacterial, fungal, and malarial parasites' whole genome information [41–43]. These algorithms are used in predicting vaccine candidates, for example, in the integrated approach used by Pritam et al. [44]. In contrast to the approaches used in other facets of infectious disease research, vaccine research uses an integrated approach by considering the prediction of antigenicity, epitope prediction, allergen prediction, and virulence prediction. Additionally, predictions of cytokine production are recommended. Many of these prediction algorithms use machine learning tools as their engines. These prediction analyses use whole-genome information regarding the total encoded proteins. Xu et al. [45] used the random forest model to predict severe asthma exacerbation in Caucasian children. They used a training dataset with 417 samples and a test dataset with 164 samples and 160 SNPs in or near 140 genes. They could obtain a sensitivity of 0.66 and a specificity of 0.6. By adjusting the threshold, a suitable sensitivity and specificity could be attained. Asthma is a complex disease with many genetic factors underlying its development. Further, the small sample sizes pose a challenge in obtaining sufficient statistical power. This experience is notable because artificial intelligence can integrate many weak predictors into a reliable predictor.

Using patient and genomic features, in 2021, some scientist have [46] used machine-learning tools to predict Carbapenem-resistant *Klebsiella pneumoniae* (CRKP). Although the aim was approached from very different data, the prediction accuracy was similar between the patient and the genomic features. The patient's features included duration of stay and kidney diseases. The genomic features included mobile genetic elements and disruption in the O-antigen gene structure. The O-antigen disruption increased its association with the respiratory tract, meaning that changes in this gene could confer the ability to evade the immune system. Further, acquiring the mobile genetic element with virulent factors such as yersiniabactin and colibactin confers increased virulence. Many antibiotic-resistant determinants encoded by antibiotic-resistance genes were associated with colonization. This revelation during the usage of machine learning tools is an example of generating a new understanding of the dynamics of genetic changes in pathogens. Such dynamics can be uncovered through genomics sequencing and rapidly identified through artificial intelligence, thereby opening a new understanding of treatments. Identifying variants from genomic sequence data is a priority in healthcare for diagnosing diseases in individuals with an underlying genetic variation. After sequencing, the steps involved are alignment to a reference genome, variant calling, variant annotation, prioritization, and diagnosis [47]. Friedman et al. [48] used convolutional neural networks to improve the sensitivity and precision of variant calls and published a new tool, *CNNS core variants.* Recently, NVIDIA developed *NVScoreVariants, a variant* of the original tool, *CNNScoreVariants* [49]. NVIDIA has also developed Clara Parabricks for genomics data analysis. This suite of multiple analytical workflows uses a graphics processing unit (GPU) environment with speed enhancement. Speed and high accuracy are of the essence when using genomics data. The NVIDIA architecture is a game-changer in this direction. GPUs have parallel processing capabilities and high memory bandwidth.

Poplin et al. published the DeepVariant software for universal SNP and small-indel variant calling using deep neural networks [50]. It uses a deep convolutional neural network on aligned Next-Generation Sequencing

(NGS) reads and the candidate variant sites where the read pileup images are calculated for their genotype likelihoods. This product was developed as a collaboration between Verily Life Sciences and Google Inc. DeepVariant can call variants from a variety of data from various sequencing technologies. DeepTrio is built on DeepVariant and considers the variants of the mother-father-child trio [51]. The fact that a genomics team is set in Google Health is testimony to the use of genomics in healthcare along with state-of-the-art methods of artificial intelligence.

## 8.10 IMPACT OF AI ON GENOMICS

AI helps assemble the vast amounts of data generated from genomics experiments, and investigators can gain near-accurate pictures of biological systems. Secondly, hypothesis-based research experiments are replaced by analyzing the datasets without prior assumptions using AI tools. Further, this type of study increases the chances of winning a research grant. AI shortens the time of genome sequencing and reduces errors. It also helps identify variants. Personalizing medications is another area where AI has a significant impact and enhances scalability. This generation has a historic opportunity and responsibility to transform medicine by using systematic approaches in the biological sciences to dramatically accelerate the understanding and treatment of disease [52].

## 8.11 LIMITATIONS OF AI

AI applications can lead to unethical and discriminatory circumstances and thus may raise regulatory issues. AI methods have to be carefully monitored and tested, as they can have serious implications for human health. Data privacy could be a challenge. The cost and expertise required to deploy AI algorithms also increase with the increase in biomedical data. AI has limitations in generating human-readable predictions along with reasoning. Machines could be biased toward certain diseases and populations. AI requires continuous training on existing datasets.

## 8.12 ETHICAL ASPECTS OF THE USE OF AI IN THE AREA OF GENOMICS

AI is designed to consider only the potential benefits of early disclosure of incidental findings for the fetus or the potential benefit for the parents in having this information, such as for their health. They might want to know if some early intervention could ameliorate the unrelated condition. While the possibility and implications of returning incidental findings should be discussed before an ultrasound is conducted, in some cases, these questions will only occur to parents after a result has been returned.

AI could play a role in scaling up risks. Research shows, for example, that AI can increase overdiagnosis [53]. AI may identify many additional variants associated with genetic disease that lack a definitive causative effect or may not be associated with clinical benefit. This could cause unnecessary anxiety and distress for parents. Consider the detection of variants in the fetus that predispose adults to develop breast cancer when a majority will either never develop tumors or develop them at the limitations of AI.

AI applications can lead to unethical and discriminatory circumstances and thus may raise regulatory issues. AI methods have to be carefully monitored and tested as they can have serious implications for human health. Data privacy could be a challenge. The cost and expertise required to deploy AI algorithms increase with increased biomedical data. AI has a limitation in generating human-readable predictions along with reasoning. Machines could be biased toward certain diseases and populations. AI requires continuous training on existing datasets.

A life stage may exist where treatment is not beneficial. Prenatal detection could prompt parents to consider terminating their pregnancy based on a dubious cancer risk.

Another important ethical issue concerns data privacy and security within AI systems trained on copious sensitive data. Analysis of current prenatal cases will be most effective when there are large amounts of data from previous cases to compare with, provided the information about the clinical picture of the fetus (e.g., what the fetal abnormalities are) is linked to the genomic data. This becomes important for ultra-rare conditions where individuals are particularly identifiable.

It has been argued that we should not disclose certain genetic test results when they pose significant risks to fetal privacy [54]. These considerations are especially relevant in the case of ultra-rare conditions. However, genomic data from individuals with ultra-rare conditions will be an especially valuable resource when linked to clinical information and would be highly sought after by pharmaceutical and insurance companies.

## 8.13 FUTURE DIRECTIONS

AI continues to evolve rapidly, with ongoing efforts to develop more advanced algorithms capable of handling increasingly complex biological data. Interdisciplinary collaborations among computer scientists, biologists, and clinicians drive innovation in single-cell sequencing, metagenomics, and systems biology. AI is also being applied to address challenges in drug discovery, such as drug repurposing, target identification, and virtual screening of compound libraries. Overall, AI has become indispensable in life sciences, revolutionizing how we study, understand, and apply biological information to improve human health and address societal challenges.

## REFERENCES


1. "A Brief History of Artificial Intelligence: On the Past, Present, and Future of Artificial Intelligence - Michael Haenlein, Andreas Kaplan, 2019." Retrieved 30 July 2024. https://journals.sagepub.com/doi/10.1177/0008125619864925
2. Bhardwaj, A., Kishore, S., and Pandey, D. K., "Artificial Intelligence in Biological Sciences," *Life*, Vol. 12, No. 9, 2022, p. 1430. https://doi.org/10.3390/life12091430
3. Xu, Y., Liu, X., Cao, X., Huang, C., Liu, E., Qian, S., Liu, X., Wu, Y., Dong, F., Qiu, C.-W., Qiu, J., Hua, K., Su, W., Wu, J., Xu, H., Han, Y., Fu, C., Yin, Z., Liu, M., Roepman, R., Dietmann, S., Virta, M., Kengara, F., Zhang, Z., Zhang, L., Zhao, T., Dai, J., Yang, J., Lan, L., Luo, M., Liu, Z., An, T., Zhang, B., He, X., Cong, S., Liu, X., Zhang, W., Lewis, J. P., Tiedje, J. M., Wang, Q., An, Z., Wang, F., Zhang, L., Huang, T., Lu, C., Cai, Z., Wang, F., and Zhang, J., "Artificial Intelligence: A Powerful Paradigm for Scientific Research," *The Innovation*, Vol. 2, No. 4, 2021. https://doi.org/10.1016/j.xinn.2021.100179
4. McCulloch, W. S., and Pitts, W., "A Logical Calculus of the Ideas Immanent in Nervous Activity," *The bulletin of mathematical biophysics*, Vol. 5, No. 4, 1943, pp. 115–133. https://doi.org/10.1007/BF02478259
5. Rosenblatt, F., "The Perceptron: A Probabilistic Model for Information Storage and Organization in the Brain," *Psychological Review*, Vol. 65, No. 6, 1958, pp. 386–408. https://doi.org/10.1037/h0042519
6. Hubel, D. H., and Wiesel, T. N., "Receptive Fields, Binocular Interaction and Functional Architecture in the Cat's Visual Cortex," *The Journal of Physiology*, Vol. 160, No. 1, 1962, pp. 106-154.2.
7. Fukushima, K., "Neocognitron: A Self-Organizing Neural Network Model for a Mechanism of Pattern Recognition Unaffected by Shift in Position," *Biological Cybernetics*, Vol. 36, No. 4, 1980, pp. 193–202. https://doi.org/10.1007/BF00344251
8. Kurakin, G., "How AI Originates from Biology – and How It Returns to It," *The Biochemist*, Vol. 46, No. 2, 2024, pp. 3–6. https://doi.org/10.1042/bio_2024_120
9. November, J. A., *Digitizing Life: The Introduction of Computers to Biology and Medicine*, Princeton University, 2006.
10. Buchanan, B. G., "Oral History Interview with Bruce G. Buchanan," 1991. Retrieved 1 August 2024. https://hdl.handle.net/11299/107165
11. Shortliffe, E. H., "Mycin: A Knowledge-Based Computer Program Applied to Infectious Diseases," *Proceedings of the Annual Symposium on Computer Application in Medical Care*, 1977, pp. 66–69.
12. Stormo, G. D., Schneider, T. D., Gold, L., and Ehrenfeucht, A., "Use of the 'Perceptron' Algorithm to Distinguish Translational Initiation Sites in E. Coli," *Nucleic Acids Research*, Vol. 10, No. 9, 1982, pp. 2997–3011. https://doi.org/10.1093/nar/10.9.2997

13. Churchill, G. A., "Hidden Markov Chains and the Analysis of Genome Structure," *Computers and Chemistry*, Vol. 16, No. 2, 1992, pp. 107–115.
14. Yang, A., Zhang, W., Wang, J., Yang, K., Han, Y., and Zhang, L., "Review on the Application of Machine Learning Algorithms in the Sequence Data Mining of DNA," *Frontiers in Bioengineering and Biotechnology*, Vol. 8, 2020. https://doi.org/10.3389/fbioe.2020.01032
15. Mittal, S., Jena, M. K., and Pathak, B., "Machine Learning Empowered next Generation DNA Sequencing: Perspective and Prospectus," *Chemical Science*, 2024. https://doi.org/10.1039/D4SC01714E
16. Alipanahi, B., Delong, A., Weirauch, M. T., and Frey, B. J., "Predicting the Sequence Specificities of DNA- and RNA-Binding Proteins by Deep Learning," *Nature Biotechnology*, Vol. 33, No. 8, 2015, pp. 831–838. https://doi.org/10.1038/nbt.3300
17. Zhou, J., and Troyanskaya, O. G., "Predicting Effects of Noncoding Variants with Deep Learning–Based Sequence Model," *Nature Methods*, Vol. 12, No. 10, 2015, pp. 931–934. https://doi.org/10.1038/nmeth.3547
18. Yandell, M. D., and Majoros, W. H., "Genomics and Natural Language Processing," *Nature Reviews Genetics*, Vol. 3, No. 8, 2002, pp. 601–610. https://doi.org/10.1038/nrg861
19. Katsura, Y., et.al.., "The Landscape of Tolerated Genetic Variation in Humans and Primates," *Science (New York, N.Y.)*, Vol. 380, No. 6648, 2023, p. eabn8153. https://doi.org/10.1126/science.abn8197
20. Jia, X., Yang, L., Li, C., Xu, Y., Yang, Q., and Chen, F., "Combining Comparative Genomic Analysis with Machine Learning Reveals Some Promising Diagnostic Markers to Identify Five Common Pathogenic Non-tuberculous Mycobacteria," *Microbial Biotechnology*, Vol. 14, No. 4, 2021, pp. 1539–1549. https://doi.org/10.1111/1751-7915.13815
21. Azouri, D., Abadi, S., Mansour, Y., Mayrose, I., and Pupko, T., "Harnessing Machine Learning to Guide Phylogenetic-Tree Search Algorithms," *Nature Communications*, Vol. 12, No. 1, 2021, p. 1983. https://doi.org/10.1038/s41467-021-22073-8
22. Rees, H. A., and Liu, D. R., "Base Editing: Precision Chemistry on the Genome and Transcriptome of Living Cells," *Nature Reviews. Genetics*, Vol. 19, No. 12, 2018, pp. 770–788. https://doi.org/10.1038/s41576-018-0059-1
23. Yan, J., Cirincione, A., and Adamson, B., "Prime Editing: Precision Genome Editing by Reverse Transcription," *Molecular Cell*, Vol. 77, No. 2, 2020, pp. 210–212. https://doi.org/10.1016/j.molcel.2019.12.016
24. Dixit, S., Kumar, A., Srinivasan, K., Vincent, P. M. D. R., and Ramu Krishnan, N., "Advancing Genome Editing with Artificial Intelligence: Opportunities, Challenges, and Future Directions," *Frontiers in Bioengineering and Biotechnology*, Vol. 11, 2024. https://doi.org/10.3389/fbioe.2023.1335901
25. Huang, J., Lin, Q., Fei, H., He, Z., Xu, H., Li, Y., Qu, K., Han, P., Gao, Q., Li, B., Liu, G., Zhang, L., Hu, J., Zhang, R., Zuo, E., Luo, Y., Ran, Y., Qiu, J.-L., Zhao, K. T., and Gao, C., "Discovery of Deaminase Functions by Structure-Based Protein Clustering," *Cell*, Vol. 186, No. 15, 2023, pp. 3182–3195.e14. https://doi.org/10.1016/j.cell.2023.05.041
26. Bryant, P., "Deep Learning for Protein Complex Structure Prediction," *Current Opinion in Structural Biology*, Vol. 79, 2023, p. 102529. https://doi.org/10.1016/j.sbi.2023.102529

27. Ruffolo, J. A., Chu, L.-S., Mahajan, S. P., and Gray, J. J., "Fast, Accurate Antibody Structure Prediction from Deep Learning on Massive Set of Natural Antibodies," *Nature Communications*, Vol. 14, 2023, p. 2389. https://doi.org/10.1038/s41467-023-38063-x
28. Baek, M., DiMaio, F., Anishchenko, I., Dauparas, J., Ovchinnikov, S., Lee, G. R., Wang, J., Cong, Q., Kinch, L. N., Schaeffer, R. D., Millán, C., Park, H., Adams, C., Glassman, C. R., DeGiovanni, A., Pereira, J. H., Rodrigues, A. V., van Dijk, A. A., Ebrecht, A. C., Opperman, D. J., Sagmeister, T., Buhlheller, C., Pavkov-Keller, T., Rathinaswamy, M. K., Dalwadi, U., Yip, C. K., Burke, J. E., Garcia, K. C., Grishin, N. V., Adams, P. D., Read, R. J., and Baker, D., "Accurate Prediction of Protein Structures and Interactions Using a Three-Track Neural Network," *Science (New York, N.Y.)*, Vol. 373, No. 6557, 2021, pp. 871–876. https://doi.org/10.1126/science.abj8754
29. Terwilliger, T. C., Liebschner, D., Croll, T. I., Williams, C. J., McCoy, A. J., Poon, B. K., Afonine, P. V., Oeffner, R. D., Richardson, J. S., Read, R. J., and Adams, P. D., "AlphaFold Predictions Are Valuable Hypotheses and Accelerate but Do Not Replace Experimental Structure Determination," *Nature Methods*, Vol. 21, No. 1, 2024, pp. 110–116. https://doi.org/10.1038/s41592-023-02087-4
30. García-Giménez, J. L., Sanchis-Gomar, F., Lippi, G., Mena, S., Ivars, D., Gomez-Cabrera, M. C., Viña, J., and Pallardó, F. V., "Epigenetic Biomarkers: A New Perspective in Laboratory Diagnostics," *Clinica Chimica Acta; International Journal of Clinical Chemistry*, Vol. 413, Nos. 19–20, 2012, pp. 1576–1582. https://doi.org/10.1016/j.cca.2012.05.021
31. Mathieu, A., Leclercq, M., Sanabria, M., Perin, O., and Droit, A., "Machine Learning and Deep Learning Applications in Metagenomic Taxonomy and Functional Annotation," *Frontiers in Microbiology*, Vol. 13, 2022. https://doi.org/10.3389/fmicb.2022.811495
32. Zaman, S. B., Hussain, M. A., Nye, R., Mehta, V., Mamun, K. T., and Hossain, N., "A Review on Antibiotic Resistance: Alarm Bells Are Ringing," *Cureus*, Vol. 9, No. 6, 2017, p. e1403. https://doi.org/10.7759/cureus.1403
33. Nathan, C., "Resisting Antimicrobial Resistance," *Nature Reviews. Microbiology*, Vol. 18, No. 5, 2020, pp. 259–260. https://doi.org/10.1038/s41579-020-0348-5
34. Wani, A. K., Roy, P., Kumar, V., and Mir, T. ul G., "Metagenomics and Artificial Intelligence in the Context of Human Health," *Infection, Genetics and Evolution*, Vol. 100, 2022, p. 105267. https://doi.org/10.1016/j.meegid.2022.105267
35. Franzosa, E. A., Huang, K., Meadow, J. F., Gevers, D., Lemon, K. P., Bohannan, B. J. M., and Huttenhower, C., "Identifying Personal Microbiomes Using Metagenomic Codes," *Proceedings of the National Academy of Sciences of the United States of America*, Vol. 112, No. 22, 2015, pp. E2930-2938. https://doi.org/10.1073/pnas.1423854112
36. Yang, J., Tsukimi, T., Yoshikawa, M., Suzuki, K., Takeda, T., Tomita, M., and Fukuda, S., "Cutibacterium Acnes (Propionibacterium Acnes) 16S rRNA Genotyping of Microbial Samples from Possessions Contributes to Owner Identification," *mSystems*, Vol. 4, No. 6, 2019, p. 10.1128/msystems.00594-19. https://doi.org/10.1128/msystems.00594-19

37. Lopez-Rincon, A., Tonda, A., Mendoza-Maldonado, L., Mulders, D. G. J. C., Molenkamp, R., Perez-Romero, C. A., Claassen, E., Garssen, J., and Kraneveld, A. D., "Classification and Specific Primer Design for Accurate Detection of SARS-CoV-2 Using Deep Learning," *Scientific Reports*, Vol. 11, No. 1, 2021, p. 947. https://doi.org/10.1038/s41598-020-80363-5
38. "Whole-Genome Sequencing Surveillance and Machine Learning of the Electronic Health Record for Enhanced Healthcare Outbreak Detection | Clinical Infectious Diseases | Oxford Academic." Retrieved 28 November 2024. https://academic.oup.com/cid/article/75/3/476/6425830
39. "A Schema for Digitized Surface Swab Site Metadata in Open-Source DNA Sequence Databases | mSystems." Retrieved 28 November 2024. https://journals.asm.org/doi/10.1128/msystems.01284-22
40. "Biological Machine Learning Combined with Campylobacter Population Genomics Reveals Virulence Gene Allelic Variants Cause Disease." Retrieved 29 November 2024. https://www.mdpi.com/2076-2607/8/4/549
41. "SPAAN: A Software Program for Prediction of Adhesins and Adhesin-like Proteins Using Neural Networks | Bioinformatics | Oxford Academic." Retrieved 29 November 2024. https://academic.oup.com/bioinformatics/article/21/4/483/203282
42. Ansari, F. A., Kumar, N., Bala Subramanyam, M., Gnanamani, M., and Ramachandran, S., "MAAP: Malarial Adhesins and Adhesin-like Proteins Predictor," *Proteins: Structure, Function, and Bioinformatics*, Vol. 70, No. 3, 2008, pp. 659–666. https://doi.org/10.1002/prot.21568
43. Chaudhuri, R., Ansari, F. A., Raghunandanan, M. V., and Ramachandran, S., "FungalRV: Adhesin Prediction and Immunoinformatics Portal for Human Fungal Pathogens," *BMC Genomics*, Vol. 12, No. 1, 2011, p. 192. https://doi.org/10.1186/1471-2164-12-192
44. Pritam, M., Singh, G., Swaroop, S., Singh, A. K., and Singh, S. P., "Exploitation of Reverse Vaccinology and Immunoinformatics as Promising Platform for Genome-Wide Screening of New Effective Vaccine Candidates against Plasmodium Falciparum," *BMC Bioinformatics*, Vol. 19, No. 13, 2019, p. 468. https://doi.org/10.1186/s12859-018-2482-x
45. Xu, M., Tantisira, K. G., Wu, A., Litonjua, A. A., Chu, J., Himes, B. E., Damask, A., and Weiss, S. T., "Genome Wide Association Study to Predict Severe Asthma Exacerbations in Children Using Random Forests Classifiers," *BMC Medical Genetics*, Vol. 12, No. 1, 2011, p. 90. https://doi.org/10.1186/1471-2350-12-90
46. "Patient and Microbial Genomic Factors Associated with Carbapenem-Resistant *Klebsiella pneumoniae* Extraintestinal Colonization and Infection | mSystems." Retrieved 29 November 2024. https://journals.asm.org/doi/10.1128/msystems.00177-21
47. Gorzynski, J. E., et.al., "Ultrarapid Nanopore Genome Sequencing in a Critical Care Setting," *New England Journal of Medicine*, Vol. 386, No. 7, 2022, pp. 700–702. https://doi.org/10.1056/NEJMc2112090
48. Friedman, S., Gauthier, L., Farjoun, Y., and Banks, E., "Lean and Deep Models for More Accurate Filtering of SNP and INDEL Variant Calls," *Bioinformatics*, Vol. 36, No. 7, 2020, pp. 2060–2067. https://doi.org/10.1093/bioinformatics/btz901

49. "Introducing NVIDIA's NVScoreVariants, a New Deep Learning Tool for Filtering Variants," GATK, Jul 01 2024. Retrieved 29 November 2024. https://gatk.broadinstitute.org/hc/en-us/articles/10064202674971-Introducing-NVIDIA-s-NVScoreVariants-a-new-deep-learning-tool-for-filtering-variants
50. Poplin, R., Chang, P.-C., Alexander, D., Schwartz, S., Colthurst, T., Ku, A., Newburger, D., Dijamco, J., Nguyen, N., Afshar, P. T., Gross, S. S., Dorfman, L., McLean, C. Y., and DePristo, M. A., "A Universal SNP and Small-Indel Variant Caller Using Deep Neural Networks," *Nature Biotechnology*, Vol. 36, No. 10, 2018, pp. 983–987. https://doi.org/10.1038/nbt.4235
51. "Analyzing Genomic Data in Families with Deep Learning," Google Open Source Blog. Retrieved 29 November 2024. https://opensource.googleblog.com/2021/04/analyzing-genomic-data-in-families-with-deep-learning.html
52. Vilhekar, R. S., and Rawekar, A., "Artificial Intelligence in Genetics," *Cureus*, Vol. 16, No. 1, p. e52035. https://doi.org/10.7759/cureus.52035
53. "Immunogenicity of the Ad26.COV2.S Vaccine for COVID-19 | Vaccination | JAMA | JAMA Network." Retrieved 28 November 2024. https://jamanetwork.com/journals/jama/fullarticle/2777598
54. Botkin, J. R., "Fetal Privacy and Confidentiality," *The Hastings Center Report*, Vol. 25, No. 5, 1995, pp. 32–39. https://doi.org/10.2307/3562793

Chapter 9

# Trends and challenges in the field of medical sciences using AI

*Rashmi Rameshwari, Sonia Kaushik, Srinivasan Ramachandran, Devendra Kumar Verma, and Santosh Kumar*

## 9.1 INTRODUCTION

Artificial intelligence (AI) has a rich history that spans several decades. Initially described by Alan Turing in 1950, AI has experienced periods of rapid advancement and stagnation, often referred to as "AI winters."[1] Since then, AI has evolved significantly, leading to breakthroughs in various fields, including medicine. Some of the earliest work in applied AI dealt with biomedicine. In the 1950s, AI was first described, but limitations in early models hindered its widespread acceptance and application in medicine.[2] In 1964, Joseph Weizenbaum created the first social robot Eliza, which communicated using pattern matching and substitution algorithms, laying the foundation for today's chatbots.[3] In 1972, MYCIN, an AI system, was developed using backward chaining. In 1986, researchers developed Dxplain, which initially handled only 500 illness problems. Over time, it expanded to cover more than 2,400 illness types. During the subsequent two decades, there was no significant use of AI in medicine. In the early 2000s, deep learning techniques emerged, overcoming many limitations faced by earlier models. These advances allowed AI to take a significant step forward in medical reasoning and medical diagnosis interpretation. Researchers explored various applications, including expert systems, data science, and machine learning (ML). However, in 2007, IBM introduced Watson, a question-answering system, which sparked renewed interest in AI within the medical community (Table 9.1).

However, over time, advances in computing and communication technologies paved the way for medical AI to evolve. Medical AI has since grown, driven by improvements in hardware and the increasing availability of labeled data. It has found applications in personalized medicine, community health, protection, medical education, and virtual care.[4] Synergies between AI and cognitive science have also influenced Artificial Intelligence and Machine Learning (AIM) research. To anticipate its further evolution, we must combine recent advances with lessons learned from the last four decades. The journey of AI in medicine continues, promising innovative solutions for healthcare.

DOI: 10.1201/9781003741770-9

*Table 9.1* The journey of AI in medicine

| *Year* | *Event* |
|---|---|
| 1950 | Alan Turing developed the "Turing Test" |
| 1952 | Machine learning |
| 1956 | John McCarthy coined the term "AI" |
| 1961 | Unimate, the first industrial robot, joined the assembly line at GM |
| 1964 | First chatbot—Eliza |
| 1966 | First electronic person—Shakey |
| 1972 | MYCIN developed |
| 1973 | SUMEX-AIM created |
| 1975 | The first NIH-sponsored AIM workshop held |
| 1980 | Development of EMYCIN—expert rule-based system |
| 1986 | Release of Dxplain—a decision support system |
| 2000 | Deep learning |
| 2007 | IBM began development of DeepQA technology (WATSON) |
| 2010 | CAD applied to endoscopy |
| 2011 | Apple's Virtual Assistant SIRI is integrated into iPhones |
| 2014 | Amazon's Virtual Assistant ALEXA is released |
| 2015 | Pharmbot was built |
| 2017 | Chatbot MANDY—automated patient intake |
| 2017 | ARTERYS—First FDA-approved cloud-based DL application in healthcare |
| 2018 | AI trials in gastroenterology |
| 2020 | Unsupervised learning |
| 2022 | GenAI |
| 2023 | ChatGPT released |
| 2024 | Microsoft Copilot released |

## 9.2 CURRENT TRENDS

AI pertains to the creation of algorithms intended to execute tasks usually performed by humans, exhibiting intelligent behavior. Currently, there is renewed interest in AI, driven by significant advances in computing power and data generation. High-tech companies have achieved remarkable successes in areas such as game playing, visual identification, and understanding of human language, machine translation, and self-driving cars.

## 9.3 AI APPLICATIONS IN RECOGNITION, PROBLEM-SOLVING, AND PATIENT CARE

In the realm of diagnostics, AI is widely used in the healthcare industry. Integrating AI into healthcare systems, precision medicine becomes increasingly feasible, allowing for targeted and individualized therapies. AI's ability to rapidly process vast amounts of healthcare information with unmatched precision is a significant contribution to the healthcare industry. Unlike conventional diagnostic methods that rely on manual interpretation, AI systems excel at deciphering complex datasets, identifying patterns, and drawing relevant conclusions. This leads to faster and more precise illness identification in diagnostics.[5]

Artificial intelligence (AI) is revolutionizing medical imaging, particularly through innovations like computer vision. Deep learning algorithms can meticulously analyze images from magnetic resonance imaging (MRI), computed tomography (CT) scans, and X-rays, often surpassing human expertise. This advancement enhances early disease diagnosis, including cancers, heart disease, and mental disorders, while even expediting the diagnostic process. In digital imaging, AI is showing advancement in pathology. Pathologists employ AI algorithms to analyze tissue samples and identify patterns that may indicate various diseases. This expedites the diagnostic procedure and enhances reliability by reducing errors. AI plays an essential role in medical diagnostics.

### 9.3.1 Medical imaging interpretation

Radiologists and pathologists routinely analyze digital images to guide treatment and contribute to research. The assessments made by radiologists and pathologists directly influence clinical decisions, guiding patient treatment and predicting outcomes. Precision medicine is an evolving healthcare approach that increases the diagnosis and treatment process, leading to individual treatment and therapy planning for individual patients.[6] In the evolving landscape of precision medicine, physicians now rely more than ever on sophisticated molecular and genomic tests. These advanced diagnostic tools complement standard pathology and clinical radiology practices, enabling refined patient stratification and personalized care management. Recent breakthroughs in digital imaging, genomic medicine, and outstanding computation facilitate concurrent consideration of various clinico-pathologic information. These advancements offer unprecedented insights into the given process of illness roadmap and pave the way for developing a new way of prediction.

AI algorithms analyze images from MRI, CT scans, and X-rays with high precision, often surpassing human experts. This aids in early disease detection, including conditions like cancer, heart disease, and neurological disorders.[7]

Computer vision innovations transform how radiological scans are interpreted, ensuring consistent and reliable results.

Pathologists use AI algorithms to analyze tissue samples. These algorithms identify patterns that could indicate different diseases, assisting pathologists in their diagnostic work[8] (Table 9.2).

*Table 9.2* Therapeutic areas vs the AI method applied over the years by different research groups

| S. no. | *Disease area* | *AI method/technique* | *Accuracy/result* | *References* |
|---|---|---|---|---|
| 1 | Alzheimer | SVM, a decision tree algorithm | Less than 90% accuracy | 9 |
| 2 | Cardiac arrest | Machine learning, KNN, IoT | Accuracy: 96% | 10 |
| 3 | The circulatory system or blood-vascular system | Algorithms like RF, DT, LRS vector machine, and KNN | Less than 86% accuracy | |
| 4 | COVID-19 | CNN | 94% accuracy | 11 |
| 5 | Hypertension and diabetes | DPM | 96.74% accuracy | 12 |
| 6 | Detection of stroke due to large artery occlusion | LVO algorithm | Less than 93% sensitivity | 13 |
| 7 | Leukemia cancer | Support vector machine, K-nearest neighbors, Naïve Bayes, and C4.5DT algorithms | Accuracy of classification and performance on microarray datasets surpass those of other individual classifiers | 14 |
| 8 | Liver disease | ANN model | Accuracy: 99% | 15 |
| 9 | Liver cirrhosis | Most of the useful and accurate algorithms: RF, multilayer perceptron, and LR | Less than 99% of accuracy | 16 |
| 10 | Lung cancer | SVM, random forest, and ANN algorithms | Less than 98% of accuracy | 17 |
| 11 | Prostatic adenocarcinoma | Support vector machine, DT, multilayer perceptron | 99.06% accuracy of model | 18 |
| 12 | Retinopathy detection | Digital imaging software | Less than 91% of sensitivity, and less than 76% of specificity | 19 |
| 13 | Skin cancer | SVM and KNN | Less than 98% accuracy | 20 |
| 14 | Skin disease | MLP and ANN | Up to 77% of accuracy | 21 |
| 15 | Thyroid illness | ANN, RF, and MP | Up to 99% accuracy | 22 |
| 16 | Thyroidal illness | KNN and SVM | Up to 85% accuracy | 23 |
| 17 | Tuberculosis | RF and ANN | Up to 89% accuracy | 24 |
| 18 | Type 1 diabetes | RF | 0.80—AUC | 25 |
| 19 | Longitudinal root fracture | CNN, DN | Up to 0.94 precise | 26 |

## 9.3.2 Disease progression prediction

AI models determine illness pathways, diagnosis, treatment processes, and possible high-risk alerts that are obtained from electronic health records (EHRs) and other sources (Figure 9.1). These models assist medical services in obtaining well-believed results and treatment plans for individual needs. Predictive modeling is a sophisticated process that uses top-level computational and digital methods to predict future events. While this tool has numerous applications in medicine, its full potential within the field remains largely untapped.[9]

Mauro F. Pinto and team investigated the potential of using ML techniques to determine the progression of multiple sclerosis. The method simulates a real medical environment effectively by utilizing all data to train a model. This model is then fit for testing any ill person. Continuing from this, it offers a comprehensive analysis of illness advancement by accumulating information over consecutive years. This approach provides a unique perspective on the evolving importance and performance of various predictors.[10]

As of November 22, 2020, more than 180 nations had documented a cumulative approximate of 57 million fixed cases of COVID-19. Numerous studies have analyzed key factors contributing to disease progression and medical diagnosis, identifying age and immune response as potential risk factors. The scientists have created an ML-based prediction for disease progression. Clinical characteristics, white blood cell count, biomarker, liver function, nephritic and kidney function, and congealing were compiled and used to set up the predictive analytic model. The predictive models, established using ML, demonstrated clear effectiveness in predicting illness progress for these subsets.[11]

Illnesses in multifaceted mind conditions significantly affect large populations globally, making investigation and medication considerably difficult. Nowadays, improvements in DL-based progress have demonstrated the capability of determining illness stages by the application of different models. The research team worked on a groundbreaking deep-learning model based on a plot depiction approach, designed to achieve extremely exact diagnostic forecasts. The study demonstrates the superiority of multimodal graph classifiers over single-modality classifiers.[12] Zhou and colleagues investigated cardiotoxicity resulting from carcinogen treatment, which increases patients' vulnerability to blood vascular system illnesses.

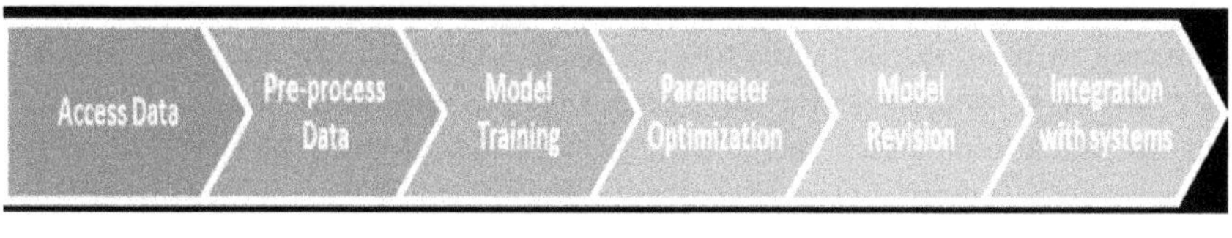


*Figure 9.1* Steps of AI model development

The study trained five different machine learning classifiers to compare their diagnostic predictions for irregular heartbeat, cardiac failure, ischemic heart disease, tissue death of heart muscle, and carcinogen diagnosis-related heart failure. The test reports, gained by the heart-oncology department, included data from 4,309 patients and comprised two groups of medical parameters: laboratory analysis and cardiac ultrasound data. On average, logistic regression emerged as the best-performing classifier across six types of illness. This method also identified parameters that take important information, thereby demonstrating greater recognition effectiveness.[13]

### 9.3.3 Drug design and growth acceleration

AI increases the rate of drug design, analyzing huge reports and determining potential drug candidates. It identifies clear targets, optimizes medicine properties, and streamlines the development process. AI has improved significantly in clinical trials. DeepMind and AlphaFold have already demonstrated a better understanding of disease processes.

AI has begun to accelerate applications across many areas for humankind, including pharmaceutical factories and labs, emerging as a primary profit company. This chapter outlines how AI can be applied across different medical fields, including drug research and formation, drug reuse, reinforcing the efficiency of pharmaceutical production, and medical studies (Figure 9.2).[14]

The method for the production and formulation of a drug requires substantial time and money, with an estimated cost of $2.8 billion. Despite this investment, nine out of ten therapeutic molecules fail Phase II medical trials and governing recommendations. Algorithms such as nearest-neighbor classifiers, random forests (RFs), support vector machines (SVMs), and deep neural networks (DNNs) are used for virtual screening (VS) based on synthesis feasibility. These algorithms can also predict in vivo activity and toxicity.[14] Guo and colleagues combined expert systems (ESs) with artificial neural networks (ANNs) to develop a hybrid system for producing direct-filling hard gelatin capsules of piroxicam, ensuring compliance with its dissolution profile specifications. The Model Expert System (MES) evaluates input parameters to make decisions and offer recommendations for formulation development. Patient dropout from clinical trials is responsible for the failure of 30% of these trials, necessitating additional recruitment efforts to complete the study and leading to significant losses of time and money. This issue can be mitigated by closely monitoring patients and assisting them in adhering to the clinical trial protocol with AI34. AiCure developed mobile software to monitor regular medication intake in patients with schizophrenia during a Phase II trial. This innovation increased patient adherence rates by 25%, ensuring the successful completion of the medical trial.[15]

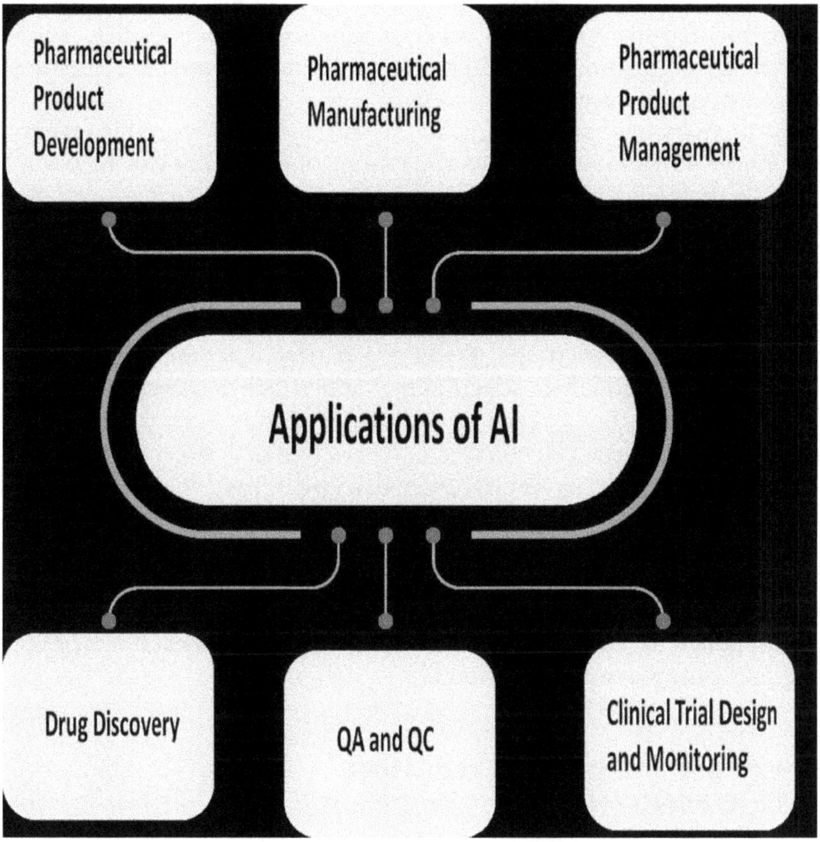


*Figure 9.2* Use of AI in various fields for the pharmaceutical area—from medicine research to product management

### 9.3.4 Remote monitoring and wearable devices

The rapid adoption of AI in medical care is transforming the field. One prevalent application is remote patient monitoring (RPM), which helps doctors oversee patients having long-standing or acute illnesses in isolated locations, senior individuals receiving domiciliary care, and even those hospitalized.[16] Scientists have explored both contact and non-contact strategies for remote patient monitoring (RPM).[17] Regardless of the type of monitoring system, all approaches focus on extracting vital signs such as heart beat, breathing frequency, systolic and diastolic pressures, and oxygen saturation, as the deterioration of these indicators impacts overall human health. Scientists have developed a diabetes determination model that classifies diabetes by incorporating not only standard factors like sugar levels, body mass index (BMI), age, and glycemic agent (insulin) but also additional external factors.[18] This study employed a variety of machine learning algorithms for diabetes prediction, such as support vector classifier, decision tree, extra tree, adaboost, neural networks, random forest, etc., boosting to enhance predictive accuracy.

Recent years have seen significant advancements in wearable technologies. These devices encompass a wide range of items that can be worn by humans, including wristwatches, glasses, chest straps, rings, and prosthetic sockets. Wearable biometric monitoring devices (BMDs) combined with artificial intelligence (AI) facilitate the real-time remote measurement and analysis of patient data. With advancements in AI, the vast amount of data collected from wearable biometric monitoring devices (BMDs) can aid in diagnosing conditions, predicting patient outcomes, and assisting healthcare professionals in selecting the most effective treatments for their patients. Scientists have introduced a creative motion-sensing system using passive radio frequency identification (RFID) tags to address the drawbacks of current elderly fall detection methods, which often rely on specialized hardware or disrupt daily life.[19] RFID technology enables motion and fall detection for elderly individuals without disrupting their daily activities. Gesture recognition and motion detection have become popular for improving human–computer interaction. In healthcare, these technologies can be applied to recognize patient gestures or movements at home or in the hospital, using a device-free system.[19]

## 9.4 POTENTIAL OF AI IN MACHINE LEARNING (ML)[5–8, 20–36]

One of the most widely used branches of AI is machine learning. Approximately 63% of American businesses have utilized AI for machine learning.[37–39]ML has been utilized in many organizational settings. Claims processing, revenue management, and record management are the areas where AI has been utilized by replacing traditional technologies. ML has been used for providing automatic warnings, pertinent information, and enhancing therapeutic procedures.[40,41] ML is basically a small group for AI; its role is to perform tasks given by data and to learn from experience, while AI may be defined as when a computer mimics human intelligence to perform tasks. Another term, "deep learning," has also been used. DL is a small group of ML by application of neural networks to solve critical problems (Table 9.3).

Major applications of ML in healthcare are as follows:

1. Personalizing treatment
2. Automatic image diagnosis
3. Drug discovery and creation
4. Assisting in clinical research

*Table 9.3* Different trends of AI for different purposes[42–48]

| *S.no.* | *Criteria* | *Class* | *Example* |
|---|---|---|---|
| 1. | Reports obtained | In language | IBM Watson, Ada, Your. MD, Gymfitty |
| | | In digital images | Third opinion, Face2Gene, Botkin AI |
| | | Report in numbers | Get In Shape, Gymfitty |
| 2. | Consumer/customer | Medico | IBM Watson, Third opinion DeepMind Health |
| | | Patient | Ada, Your.MD, Cardiio, Get In Shape, Gymfitty |
| 3. | By purpose | For diagnosis assistance | Third opinion, DeepMind Health, Face2Gene, Botkin AI |
| | | For the management of healthcare enterprises | Qventus |
| | | For a healthy body | Cardiio, Get In Shape, Gymfitty |
| | | Collecting data through inquiry | Ada, Your MD, Gymfitty |

5. Analyzing error in perceptions
6. Robot-assisted surgery
7. Detecting disease in the early stage
8. Detecting frauds
9. Identification of illness and diagnosis
10. Finding the best cure
11. Adjusting behavior
12. Medical research and diagnosis

ML is responsible for performing tasks more easily, in less time, and with reduced medical data. While ML has many applications, it also creates challenges. The medical sector has been revolutionized due to improved data analysis in less time, and accurate results also influence procedures for admin concerns in reduced time. ML helps doctors and trainees to create patients' historical disease data and to provide medications according to previous data.[59] ML is capable of performing tasks done by only humans due to its ability to adapt to new input tasks and learn from expertise. ML can also improve the medical process as it also helps prevent mistakes and error/human errors. Many diseases like tumors and cancers can be easily diagnosed with the help of AI used in ML46-49. Today, the healthcare sector would find it difficult to function without AI, and AI consulting institutions have gained significant attention in recent years. As per one study, in the United States, a 13% growth in computer-related professions has been observed in the last ten years. It does not mean that AI is the solution to all the problems. AI serves as a supportive tool for human healthcare workers and doctors. AI can function like a doctor's assistant but can never replace a doctor.

## 9.5 OPPORTUNITIES OF AI IN HEALTHCARE

It may sometimes be the case that reaching the doctor immediately is not possible; in such situations, an AI assistant becomes very helpful.[9–11, 12–14, 50–52] Engineers related to data science have now created solutions for diagnosing, possible prognosis, and also their treatment. ML can be used by using different healthcare algorithms in pathology, rare diseases, oncology, etc.

Mostly artificial ML has been utilized in neural networks. Some mobile apps on the basis of CNNs have been used, mostly in neural networks. These neural networks can be identified and recognized by the application of AI techniques. So such types of mobile apps may be very useful not only for medical facility purposes but also for academic medical colleges and institutions. For the analysis of organic fluids like blood and urine, AI in ML can be very effective in a pathologist's job, performing tasks accurately, rapidly, and repeatedly within a short time. This also creates a field of research for data scientists, as for analyzing new diseases, knowledge of different types of data analysis techniques, their interpretations, and data requirements is also a big deal.[53,54]

Now the world is looking for ML applications in healthcare. Some ML applications have attracted significant attention from the world top topmost companies for the identification of skin cancer. Stanford University researchers have detected and identified skin cancer by using DL. Cancer in mammograms has been detected by Google using AI algorithms.[55,56]

ML has been improved to a level where it can be used for the identification of illness and diagnosis. Many early-stage carcinogenic and parental illnesses, which were previously difficult to recognize, can now be identified using ML; one example is International Business Machine (IBM) Watson Genomics.[57,58] One of the AI systems developed for medical and hospital applications is PReDicT (Predicting Response to Depression Treatment).

The basic opportunities of AI in healthcare can be subdivided into five major systems:

1. Drug development
   a) Virtual screening
   b) Drug discovery
   c) Identification of potential drugs

   d) Repurposing of existing drugs
2. Diagnosis and patient monitoring
   a) Reducing healthcare costs
   b) Enabling effective patient care
   c) Medication and predictive analysis
3. Technological advancement
   a) Workflow control
   b) Decision support for clinical activities
   c) Simulation
   d) Robotic surgery and image analysis
   e) Self-monitoring
4. Virtual health assistant
   a) Patient monitoring
   b) Increase in accessibility of healthcare
   c) Providing reminders and alert systems
   d) All-time health assistance
5. Teamwork and decision-making
   a) Medical appointment maintenance
   b) Reminders and notifications regarding patient health status
   c) Communication and decision-making power
   d) Collaboration with teams as a collector

## 9.6 CHALLENGES

**Human error and data bias:** Healthcare solutions are developed using machine learning and AI systems. These systems are trained on population-derived datasets using an algorithm. It can be sensitive to data quality. Poorly labeled reports may lead to faulty findings and biased results. Deep learning algorithms, while powerful, even act like black boxes, which makes it difficult to take decisions in understanding and trust. Integrating AI into existing healthcare infrastructure and ensuring user-friendly interfaces for medical practitioners remains a significant challenge. AI-based healthcare imaging may face a data breach, providing incorrect information to doctors. This can lead to incorrect patient therapy. AI models often perform well on specific datasets derived from specific population samples. It becomes difficult to generalize across different patient groups and actual global scenarios. Due to this safety and effectiveness of AI-based healthcare is questioned. Viet-Thi Tran and team conducted a study with patients having wearable devices. Only half of the patients viewed the advancement of computational tools and AI in medicine as a significant advancement, while 11% perceived it as a threat. Although AI-based healthcare offers lots of opportunities for medical professionals, it still requires more precision to provide effective solutions to patients.

### 9.6.1 Challenges of AI in Healthcare

Challenges of AI in healthcare may be subclassified into the following points:[15–18, 50]

1. Lack of awareness of AI technology
   a) Lack of knowledge and understanding
   b) Expectations that are not realistic
2. Healthcare provider and professional liability
   c) Limited hands-on experience and practices
   d) Technology literacy level variation
   e) Professional responsibility
   f) Challenges during learning and using technology
3. Ethical and privacy-related challenges
   g) Data privacy and security
   h) Safety maintenance
   i) Transparency policies
   j) Consents for use
   k) Innovation levels for ethics
4. Unreliability of AI technology
   l) Lack of accuracy in prediction, diagnosis, and algorithms
   m) Absence of interpretation of AI algorithms and transparency
   n) Lack of coordination in model functioning
   o) Lack of sufficient clear-cut digital technology

### 9.6.2 Risk of AI in medicine

There are not only benefits to using AI in medicine, but some risks are also present. In this chapter, the authors have tried to show in short the possible risk of adopting AI. There may be seven basic risks, as shown below:

1. AI errors that can harm patients
2. Misuse of AI tools
3. Biasing with medical AI and perturbation inequality
4. Transparency issues
5. Privacy and security concerns
6. AI accountability gaps
7. Implementation in the real world

For minimizing the risks of AI and maximize its profit, it is essential to recognize, analyze, and monitor the potential risks for every new AI algorithm and its application on a case-by-case basis. For all levels of risk, they should be classified on a category basis, i.e., high risk or low risk. A set of regulations should be specified for different levels like high- or low-risk patients. For high risk, repeated testing and continuous monitoring should be performed. While it should also be kept in mind that such classification/correction should not disturb the route of health measurements and diagnosis. Some of the reasons why AI misreads are noise and artifacts in AI input and measurement. Second is shifting in data, i.e., AI obtained data and actual global reports. And the last one may be an unexpected change in clinical contents and environment. The most common biases in medical AI involve gender, age, geographical locations, and socioeconomic factors. These biases may be due to imbalanced data sheets, structural inequalities, and discriminatory data. Risk related to transparency in medical AI may be due to three main reasons: first is the difficulty in identifying the source of AI error, second is the difficulty in applying AI Algorithms and independently reproducing their results, and the third is the limited acceptance of AI systems globally. Risk for personalization and safety is also a major concern. This may occur when data is leaked or used without informing the patient or obtaining their consent. The second risk is the risk of a potential fatal cyber-attacks on AI solutions. Finally, there is risk of reusing data without the patient's knowledge.

### 9.6.3 Problems in adopting AI in India

Because of the common challenges in India and global demand for economical solutions, it has become mandatory to use AI in different fields such as agriculture, education, healthcare, transport, smart mobility, and basic construction with advanced technology. But before India adopts AI in different sectors, various challenges must be identified and addressed. India is a major producer of doctors and engineers, with quality practice and data science engineers. If we have to adopt AI in India on a large scale, some important points have to be kept in mind. First, there is an absence of collaborative efforts between stakeholders during accepting electronic health records as a kind of medical links have accepted different types of explanation of "computerized data." Second is that the related data is not present. Privacy and security policies regarding data are not uniformly understood and applied. There is a lot of chance to have anonymization of data. Lack of data ecosystem, limited AI research, especially core research in relevant technologies, shortage of AI experts and skilled manpower, low awareness of adopting by business concerns, and unclear ethical and privacy policies are complete list of challenges to adopting AI in India, but many more.

Strong determination is required for the adoption of AI in India. The Indian government can play a pivotal role in this. Funding for doing research in specified areas, financial ads from big businessmen and stakeholders need to show their interest for the adoption in India. The government can raise awareness among scientists and scholars and motivate them to do research in this area.

## 9.7 ACTION TAKEN FOR THE GOVERNMENT (RECOMMODATIONS)

Some of the strong actions should be taken by the government[59] if AI is to be adopted in India.

1. **Core research:** Setup for institutions for the center of excellence: The basic role of this center of excellence will be to find out the institutions in India, where the core research on AI can be full-fledged. For PhD scholars, a scholarship scheme or national AI fellowship should be started, so that researchers and scientists from around the world can come and collaborate. Combined projects should be started with some attractive incentives. *Interacademic collaboration*: a research collaboration between the primer institutions should be set up for the production of experts in AI, on technical basis as well as core research. *Faculty fellowship*: a combined faculty fellowship programs should be started to promote AI in different institutions, in conferences and workshops.
2. **Applied research:** Setting up of the International Centre for Transformational AI: The basic purpose of this center will be to invite expressions of interest from leading AI experts across different sectors (agriculture, healthcare, smart city projects, and education). "ICTAI Inc." should be established as a society comprising different companies. Initially it should be started with government financial support. After stabilization, a government–private partnership program can be launched.
3. **Common compute platform:** Setting up of a Big Data Analytics and Assimilation Centre that should be connected to ICTAI Inc. and all other institutions having a strong AI computing infrastructure.
4. **Intellectual property:** There should be an objective army, jointly with the Ministry of Corporate Affairs. Its role will be to examine and provide modifications in IP.
5. **Workforce:** Its work is to promote service sector jobs and employees for reskilling by training programs.
6. **Colleges and schools:** Its work will be to enhance the quality of education in the field of AI for data science and development of MOOCS programs for AI. There should be an addition as a bridge course for AI with computer engineering students and should be promotedAI in labs.
7. **Job changing:** Continuing change in the nature of jobs with skilled employees in the AI field.
8. **Awareness and adoption by government:** Demonstration of AI in workshops and conferences. To set up center–state programs for AI adoption in states.

9. **Startup support:** The government should support and provide some incentives for AI startups at a small level.
10. **Privacy and security:** A data protection framework should be set up for the protection of human rights. Research programs should be directed towards protecting and preserving privacy, while also encouraging the development of new mathematical tools, algorithms, and models to ensure robust privacy and security.
11. **Sustainable research:** Ethics, private, legal, aspects, social sustainability-related research, and study center should be developed that could also compete with world-class technologies.
12. Policy actions: The following seven strong policies should be adopted to make AI applications clinically, ethically, and technically sound.[60–65]
    a) Healthcare-specific AI regulation and policies
    b) Multi-stakeholder engagement
    c) Passwords for traceability of medical AI tools
    d) Accountability of legal frameworks
    e) Training programmers for clinical and citizens
    f) Development of strategies for the European Commission

As is well known, current AI tools/machines are regulated by Hospital Machine Regulations and the 2017/746 In Vitro Diagnostic Medical Devices Regulation (IVDR). In 2021, the European Commission proposed new regulations regarding AI in medical technologies for quality management systems and marketing monitoring policies. Thus new regulations make it tougher for the development of new AI technologies and machine/medical equipment, as they have to be more scrutinized for their use in clinical purposes.

For adoption with the least errors, professionals from the medical field will have to be trained not only to improve the medical environment and quality but also to identify areas and chance of risk. So, this is the need for updating medicine events and enhancing interdisciplinary research and study.[66–68]

## 9.8 CONCLUSION

In recent years, AI has gained popularity in healthcare and clinical and medical applications. This chapter discusses various challenges associated with applying AI for medical purposes and their various trends have been discussed. It has been observed and found that there are four types of challenges in using AI in the medical field: less knowledge of AI tools, healthcare provider and responsibility of professionals, ethical and privacy-related challenges and last one is unreliability of AI technology. It has been clearly found that AI can be highly beneficial in imaging, drug development, diagnosis and treatment, and virtual health assistance. However, patient data collection and its utilization pose significant challenges due to privacy concerns. Secondly, very few patients are aware of limited technology and professional topics. Out of the four challenges, ethical issues remain the most significant task or challenge. Public awareness and understanding also increase the mistrust and resistance to the use of AI in healthcare. With such challenges, AI also creates different powerful opportunities in five main sectors: drug development, diagnosis and patient monitoring, technological advancement, teamwork and decision-making, and virtual health assistant. AI has the potential to revolutionize medical and clinical treatment by increasing the percentage of the accuracy of diagnosis and treatment processes. However, it is critical to have actual assumptions with an ethical approach. Future research is necessary for developing standards for AI algorithms in healthcare.[16]

Some additional conclusions also arise during this chapter review. The AI use does not mean that doctors will be replaced or that they are no longer needed, nor does it replace laboratory working scientists. But this is useful for modernizing and reshaping our doctors' role. Additionally, a large public database of the human genome with strict security is needed. It is quite clear that in the future, AI will have a big role in medicine assistance, and people will also accept AI in a significant way.

## REFERENCES


1. Pandya, S., Thakur, A., Saxena, S., Jassal, N., Patel, C., Modi, K., Shah, P., Joshi, R., Gonge, S., Kadam, K., & Kadam, P. (2021). A study of the recent trends of immunology: Key challenges, domains, applications, datasets, and future directions. *Sensors*, *21*(23), 7786. https://doi.org/10.3390/s21237786
2. Shortliffe, E. H., & Shah, N. H. (2022). AI in medicine: Some pertinent history. In T. A. Cohen, V. L. Patel, & E. H. Shortliffe (Eds.), *Intelligent systems in medicine and health* (pp. 21–50). Springer International Publishing. https://doi.org/10.1007/978-3-031-09108-7_2
3. Kaul, V., Enslin, S., & Gross, S. A. (2020). History of artificial intelligence in medicine. *Gastrointestinal Endoscopy*, *92*(4), 807–812. https://doi.org/10.1016/j.gie.2020.06.040
4. Hirani, R., Noruzi, K., Khuram, H., Hussaini, A. S., Aifuwa, E. I., Ely, K. E., Lewis, J. M., Gabr, A. E., Smiley, A., Tiwari, R. K., & Etienne, M. (2024). Artificial intelligence and healthcare: A journey through history, present innovations, and future possibilities. *Life*, *14*(5), 557. https://doi.org/10.3390/life14050557
5. Olive-Gadea, M., Crespo, C., Granes, C., Hernandez-Perez, M., Pérez De La Ossa, N., Laredo, C., Urra, X., Carlos Soler, J., Soler, A., Puyalto, P., Cuadras, P., Marti, C., & Ribo, M. (2020). Deep learning based software to identify large vessel occlusion on noncontrast computed tomography. *Stroke*, *51*(10), 3133–3137. https://doi.org/10.1161/STROKEAHA.120.030326

6. Pattichis, C. S., Pitris, C., Liang, J., & Zhang, Y. (2019). Guest editorial on the special issue on integrating informatics and technology for precision medicine. *IEEE Journal of Biomedical and Health Informatics*, *23*(1), 12–13. https://doi.org/10.1109/JBHI.2018.2885877
7. Obuchowicz, R., Strzelecki, M., & Piórkowski, A. (2024). Clinical applications of artificial intelligence in medical imaging and image processing—A review. *Cancers*, *16*(10), 1870. https://doi.org/10.3390/cancers16101870
8. Kim, I., Kang, K., Song, Y., & Kim, T.-J. (2022). Application of artificial intelligence in pathology: Trends and challenges. *Diagnostics*, *12*(11), 2794. https://doi.org/10.3390/diagnostics12112794
9. Toma, M., & Wei, O. C. (2023). Predictive modeling in medicine. *Encyclopedia*, *3*, 590–601. https://doi.org/10.3390/encyclopedia3020042
10. Pinto, M. F., Oliveira, H., Batista, S., et al. (2020). Prediction of disease progression and outcomes in multiple sclerosis with machine learning. *Scientific Reports*, *10*, 21038. https://doi.org/10.1038/s41598-020-78212-6
11. Xu, F., et al. (2021). *Phytochemistry Reviews*. https://doi.org/10.1007/s11101-021-09758-0
12. Aqil, K. H., Dumpuri, P., Ram, K., & Sivaprakasam, M. (2024). Predictive modeling of Alzheimer's disease progression: Integrating temporal clinical factors and outcomes in time series forecasting. *Intelligence-Based Medicine*, *10*, 100159.
13. Zhou, Y., et al. (2020). Clinical course and risk factors for mortality of adult inpatients with COVID-19 in Wuhan, China: A retrospective cohort study. *Lancet*, *395*(10229), 1054–1062. https://doi.org/10.1016/S0140-6736(20)30566-3
14. Paul, D., Sanap, G., Shenoy, S., Kalyane, D., Kalia, K., & Tekade, R. K. (2021). Artificial intelligence in drug discovery and development. *Drug Discovery Today*, *26*(1), 80–93. https://doi.org/10.1016/j.drudis.2020.10.010
15. Mak, K. K., & Pichika, M. R. (2019). Artificial intelligence in drug development: Present status and future prospects. *Drug Discovery Today*, *24*(3), 773–780. https://doi.org/10.1016/j.drudis.2018.11.014
16. Shaik, T., Tao, X., Higgins, N., Li, L., Gururajan, R., Zhou, X., & Acharya, U. R. (2023). *WIREs Data Mining and Knowledge Discovery*, *13*, e1485. https://doi.org/10.1002/widm.1485
17. Malasinghe, L. P., Ramzan, N., & Dahal, K. (2019). Remote patient monitoring: A comprehensive study. *Journal of Ambient Intelligence and Humanized Computing*, *10*(1), 57–76. https://doi.org/10.1007/s12652-017-0598-x
18. Mujumdar, A., & Vaidehi, V. (2019). *Procedia Computer Science*, *165*, 292–299. https://doi.org/10.1016/j.procs.2020.01.047
19. Zhu, F., Xiao, B., Liu, J., Wang, B., Pan, Q., & Chen, L.-J. (2017). Exploring tag distribution in multi-reader RFID systems. *IEEE Transactions on Mobile Computing*, *16*(5), 1300–1314. https://doi.org/10.1109/TMC.2016.2591950
20. Neelaveni, J., & Devasana, G. (2020). *6th International conference on advanced computing and communication systems (ICACCS)*.
21. Kumar, N. K., Sindhu, G. S., Prashanthi, D. K., & Sulthana, A. S. (2020). *6th International conference on advanced computing and communication systems (ICACCS)* (pp. 15–21). IEEE.
22. Islam, M. Z., Islam, M. M., & Asraf, A. (2020). A combined deep CNN-LSTM network for the detection of novel coronavirus (COVID-19) using X-ray images. *Informatics in Medicine Unlocked*, *20*, 100412.

23. Fitriyani, N. L., Syafrudin, M., Alfian, G., & Rhee, J. (2019). Development of disease prediction model based on ensemble Learning approach for diabetes and hypertension. *IEEE*, 7,144777–144789. https://doi.org/10.1109/ACCESS.2019.2945129
24. Rodrigues, T., Reker, D., Schneider, P., Schneider, G., & Schneider, P. (2016). Counting on natural products for drug design. *Nature Chemistry*, *8*, 531–541. https://doi.org/10.1038/nchem.2479
25. Alrefai, N. (2019). *International Journal of Applied Engineering Research*, *14*(21), 4077–4084.
26. Musleh, M., et al. (2019). *International Journal of Academic Information Systems Research (IJAISR)*, *3*(10), 1–11.
27. Emu, M., Yan, P., & Choudhury, S. (2020). Latency aware VNF deployment at edge devices for IoT services: An artificial neural network based approach. In *2020 IEEE international conference on communications workshops (ICC Workshops)* (pp. 1–6). IEEE. https://doi.org/10.1109/ICCWorkshops49005.2020.9145242
28. Banerjee, N., & Das, S. (2020). Prediction lung cancer – in machine learning perspective. In *2020 International conference on computer science, engineering and applications (ICCSEA)* (pp. 1–5). IEEE. https://doi.org/10.1109/ICCSEA49143.2020.9132913
29. Oyewo, O. A., & Boyinbode, O. K. (2020). *International Journal of Advanced Computer Science and Applications*, *11*(3).
30. Sarao, V., Veritti, D., & Lanzetta, P. (2020). Automated diabetic retinopathy detection with two different retinal imaging devices using artificial intelligence: A comparison study. *Graefe's Archive for Clinical and Experimental Ophthalmology*, *258*, 2647–2654. https://doi.org/10.1007/s00417-020-04853-y
31. Vidya, M., & Karki, M. V. (2020). Skin cancer detection using machine learning techniques. In *2020 IEEE international conference on electronics, computing and communication technologies (CONECCT)* (pp. 1–5). IEEE. https://doi.org/10.1109/CONECCT50063.2020.9198489
32. Naseer, M., Khan, S., & Porikli, F. (2019). Local gradients smoothing: Defense against localized adversarial attacks. In *2019 IEEE winter conference on applications of computer vision (WACV)* (pp. 1300–1307). IEEE. https://doi.org/10.1109/WACV.2019.00143
33. Bhatt, D. L., Steg, P. G., Miller, M., Brinton, E. A., Jacobson, T. A., Ketchum, S. B., ... Ballantyne, C. M. (2019). Cardiovascular risk reduction with icosapent ethyl for hypertriglyceridemia. *New England Journal of Medicine*, *380*(1), 11–22.
34. Jamkhandikar, D., & Priya, N. (2020). Thyroid disease prediction using feature selection and machine learning classifiers. *The International Journal of Analytical and Experimental Modal Analysis*, *XII*(VII).
35. Lai, J., Ma, S., Wang, Y., Cai, Z., Hu, J., Wei, N., ... Hu, S. (2020). Factors associated with mental health outcomes among health care workers exposed to coronavirus disease 2019. *JAMA Network Open*, *3*(3), e203976. https://doi.org/10.1001/jamanetworkopen.2020.3976
36. Fernåndez-Edreira, D., Liñares-Blanco, J., & Fernandez-Lozano, C. (2021). Machine learning analysis of the human infant gut microbiome identifies influential species in type 1 diabetes. *Expert Systems with Applications*, *185*, 115648. https://doi.org/10.1016/j.eswa.2021.115648

37. Aqil, K. H., Dumpuri, P., Ram, K., & Sivaprakasam, M. (2024). Predictive modeling of Alzheimer's disease progression: Integrating temporal clinical factors and outcomes in time series forecasting. *Intelligence-Based Medicine, 10,* 100159. https://doi.org/10.1016/j.ibmed.2024.100159
38. Fogel, D. B. (2018). Factors associated with clinical trials that fail and opportunities for improving the likelihood of success: A review. *Contemporary Clinical Trials Communications, 11,* 156–164. https://doi.org/10.1016/j.conctc.2018.08.001
39. Kalra, G., Peng, Y., Guo, M., & Augsburger, L. L. (2002). A hybrid intelligent system for formulation of BCS Class II drugs in hard gelatin capsules. In *Proceedings of the 9th international conference on neural information processing (ICONIP '02), 4,* 1987–1991. https://doi.org/10.1109/ICONIP.2002.1199021
40. Kwiatkowski, A., Sobolewski, O., Wyłomańska, A., Sawicki, M., Zieleń, P., Druszcz, A., & Ptak, M. (2023). Development of artificial intelligence algorithms to analyse weather conditions for the prediction of cerebrovascular accidents. In H. Podbielska & M. Kapalla (Eds.), *Predictive, preventive, and personalised medicine: From bench to bedside* (Vol. 17, pp. 283–304). Springer. https://doi.org/10.1007/978-3-031-34884-6_16
41. Mak, K.-K., & Pichika, M. R. (2019). Artificial intelligence in drug development: Present status and future prospects. *Drug Discovery Today, 24*(3), 773–780. https://doi.org/10.1016/j.drudis.2018.11.014
42. Hazarika, I. (2020). Artificial intelligence: Opportunities and implications for the health workforce. *International Health, 12*(4), 241–245. https://doi.org/10.1093/inthealth/ihaa007
43. Grace, M. K., & VanHeuvelen, J. S. (2019). Occupational variation in burnout among medical staff: Evidence for the stress of higher status. *Social Science & Medicine, 232,* 199–208. https://doi.org/10.1016/j.socscimed.2019.05.007
44. Olaronke, I., & Oluwaseun, O. (2017). Big data in healthcare: Prospects, challenges and resolutions. In *Proceedings of the future technology conference (FTC 2016)* (pp. 1152–1157). https://doi.org/10.1109/FTC.2016.7821747
45. Liu, N., Chen, C. B., & Kumara, S. (2020). Semi-supervised learning algorithm for identifying high-priority drug–drug interactions through adverse event reports. *IEEE Journal of Biomedical and Health Informatics, 24*(1), 57–68. https://doi.org/10.1109/JBHI.2019.2932740
46. Lee, D. H., & Yoon, S. N. (2021). Application of artificial intelligence–based technologies in the healthcare industry: Opportunities and challenges. *International Journal of Environmental Research and Public Health, 18*(1), 271. https://doi.org/10.3390/ijerph18010271
47. Jadczyk, T., Wojakowski, W., Tendera, M., Henry, T. D., Egnaczyk, G., & Shreenivas, S. (2021). Artificial intelligence can improve patient management at the time of a pandemic: The role of voice technology. *Journal of Medical Internet Research, 23*(5), e22959. https://doi.org/10.2196/22959
48. Bohr, A., & Memarzadeh, K. (2020). The rise of artificial intelligence in healthcare applications. In *Artificial intelligence in healthcare* (pp. 25–60). https://doi.org/10.15420/cfr.2019.14
49. Malasinghe, L. P., Ramzan, N., & Dahal, K. (2019). Remote patient monitoring: A comprehensive study. *Journal of Ambient Intelligence and Humanized Computing, 10*(1), 57–76. https://doi.org/10.1007/s12652-017-0598-x

50. Fukuda, M., Inamoto, K., Shibata, N., et al. (2020). Evaluation of an artificial intelligence system for detecting vertical root fracture on panoramic radiography. *Oral Radiology, 36,* 337–343. https://doi.org/10.1007/s11282-019-00409-x
51. Aqil, K. H., Dumpuri, P., Ram, K., & Sivaprakasam, M. (2024). Predictive modeling of Alzheimer's disease progression: Integrating temporal clinical factors and outcomes in time series forecasting. *Intelligence-Based Medicine, 10,* 100159.
52. Fogel, D. B. (2018). Factors associated with clinical trials that fail and opportunities for improving the likelihood of success: A review. *Contemporary Clinical Trials Communications, 11,* 156–164. https://doi.org/10.1016/j.conctc.2018.08.001
53. Pinto, M. F., Oliveira, H., Batista, S., Cruz, L., Pinto, M., Correia, I., Martins, P., & Teixeira, C. (2020). Prediction of disease progression and outcomes in multiple sclerosis with machine learning. *Scientific Reports, 10*(1), 21038. https://doi.org/10.1038/s41598-020-78212-6
54. Pinto-Coelho, L. (2023). How artificial intelligence is shaping medical imaging technology: A survey of innovations and applications. *Bioengineering, 10*(12), 1435. https://doi.org/10.3390/bioengineering10121435
55. Shaik, T., Tao, X., Higgins, N., Li, L., Gururajan, R., Zhou, X., & Acharya, U. R. (2023). Remote patient monitoring using artificial intelligence: Current state, applications, and challenges. *WIREs Data Mining and Knowledge Discovery, 13*(2), e1485. https://doi.org/10.1002/widm.1485
56. Tran, V.-T., Riveros, C., & Ravaud, P. (2019). Patients' views of wearable devices and AI in healthcare: Findings from the ComPaRe e-cohort. *NPJ Digital Medicine*, 2(1), 53. https://doi.org/10.1038/s41746-019-0132-y
57. Zhou, Y., Hou, Y., Hussain, M., Brown, S., Budd, T., Tang, W. H. W., ... Cheng, F. (2020). Machine learning–based risk assessment for cancer therapy–related cardiac dysfunction in 4,300 longitudinal oncology patients. *Journal of the American Heart Association*, 9(23), e019628. https://doi.org/10.1161/JAHA.120.019628
58. Zhu, L., Wang, R., Wang, Z., & Yang, H. (2017). TagCare: Using RFIDs to monitor the status of the elderly living alone. *IEEE Access, 5,* 11364–11373. https://doi.org/10.1109/ACCESS.2017.2716359
59. Jeddi, Z., & Bohr, A. (2020). Remote patient monitoring using artificial intelligence. In *Artificial intelligence in healthcare* (pp. 203–234). Academic Press. https://doi.org/10.1016/B978-0-12-818438-7.00009-5
60. Gerke, S., Minssen, T., & Cohen, G. (2020). Ethical and legal challenges of artificial intelligence–driven healthcare. In *Artificial intelligence in healthcare* (pp. 295–336). Academic Press. https://doi.org/10.1016/B978-0-12-818438-7.00012-5
61. Sun, T. Q., & Medaglia, R. (2019). Mapping the challenges of artificial intelligence in the public sector: Evidence from public healthcare. *Government Information Quarterly*, 36(2), 368–383. https://doi.org/10.1016/j.giq.2018.09.008
62. Iliashenko, O., Bikkulova, Z., & Dubgorn, A. (2019). Opportunities and challenges of artificial intelligence in healthcare. *E3S Web of Conferences, 112,* 02028. https://doi.org/10.1051/e3sconf/201911002028

63. Singh, R. P., Hom, G. L., Abramoff, M. D., Campbell, J. P., & Chiang, M. F. (2020). Current challenges and barriers to real-world artificial intelligence adoption for the healthcare system, provider, and the patient. *Translational Vision Science & Technology*, 9(2), 45. https://doi.org/10.1167/tvst.9.2.45
64. Jiang, L., Wu, Z., Xu, X., Zhan, Y., Jin, X., Wang, L., & Qiu, Y. (2021). Opportunities and challenges of artificial intelligence in the medical field: Current application, emerging problems, and problem-solving strategies. *Journal of International Medical Research*, 49(3), 1–11. https://doi.org/10.1177/03000605211004297
65. Yadav, M. K., et al. (2022). *Journal of Biomolecular Structure & Dynamics.*
66. Khan, F. N., et al. A Review on Predictive Systems and Data Models for COVID-19(2021). *Surveillance Prevention Prediction & Diagnosis,* 123.
67. Galbusera, F., et al. (2019). Artificial intelligence and machine learning in spine research. *JOR Spine, 2,* e1044.
68. Weng, S. F., et al. Can machine-learning improve cardiovascular risk prediction using routine clinical data? (2017). *PLoS One*, *12,* e0174944.

Chapter 10

# A survey of clinical decision support systems

*Vinayak Gupta, Yajnaseni Dash, Dinesh Kumar, Naween Kumar, and Sudhir C. Sarangi*

## 10.1 INTRODUCTION

### 10.1.1 Background

Due to the recent focus on healthcare 4.0, where technology plays an important role, clinical decision support systems (CDSSs) have been adopted as an essential part of the healthcare system. These systems use technologies that organize themselves to help healthcare providers make clinical decisions. Due to the use of intelligent informatics, business intelligence, and analytics, CDSS plays a vital role in promoting the quality of care while reducing attempts at clinical mistakes and errors. The application of CDSS has made it possible to make high levels of systematic decision-making about clinical management and patient care, entailing the collection and processing of complex medical data. This stringent reasoning framework is at the base of current medicine and gives healthcare practitioners the necessary updated, correct, and relevant information to manage their therapies (Beeler, 2014). Therefore, CDSS plays an important role in creating the utilization of solutions for a greater, tolerable, and error-free healthcare system to embrace the culture of patient-centered care and precision medicine. Over time, there has been an increase in the complexity of medical data due to genomics, imaging, electronic health records (EHRs), and wearable devices that have made it crucial to incorporate advanced analytics and alter the method of clinical decision-making. CDSS is beneficial because of the large amounts of patient information, which combines with medical knowledge and ensures that it provides time-bound recommendations. For instance, a CDSS can allow practitioners to know about potential drug interactions, suggest various diagnostic tests, as well as recommend personalized treatment plans based on patient-specific factors. Such capabilities show that CDSS is significant in helping as well as medicating diagnostic errors, while also ensuring that the highest standards of healthcare practices being maintained (Musen, 2021). CDSSs are not only limited to resource-rich areas but also to areas where resources are constrained. In rural or underserved areas, where there is limited access to specialized care, the

 DOI: 10.1201/9781003741770-10

implementation of CDSS helps to act as a virtual consultant, which allows the present practitioners to have greater insight. This allows for democratization of the expertise and improves the healthcare quality as well as equity for the whole medical workflow.

The general structure and functioning of the clinical decision support system (CDSS) are described in detail in Figure 10.1, which shows that there is a CDSS that is proper, as well as a CDSS that includes a dashboard for the visualization of medical data analytics—being the central process of getting and analyzing the data and information to come up with the data and analytical insights necessary to underpin diagnostic and treatment decisions based on medical datasets and other contributory information from medical practitioners and machine learning algorithms as part of AI. This figure supports the idea of an AI-based CDSS by illustrating how the overall system gathers and applies data accumulated from Human

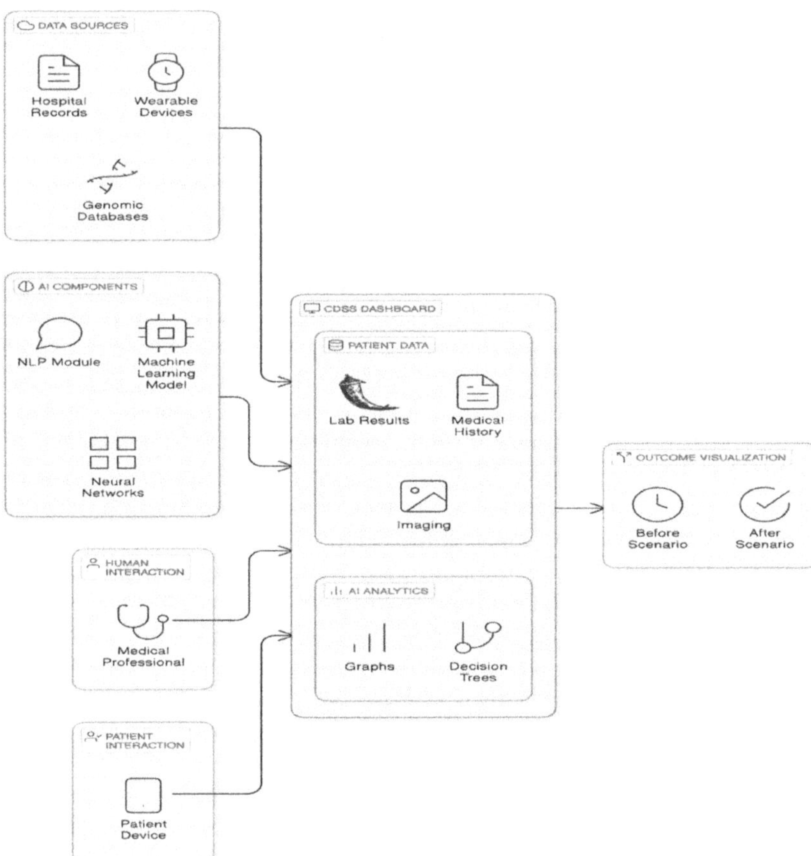


*Figure 10.1* Overflow of clinical decision support systems (CDSSs)

Intelligence (HI), Wearable Device Data (WD), and Guideline Data (GD), among others.

The system uses natural language processing equipment and machine learning options, which form part and parcel of the system's analysis. In this case, the dashboard of CDSS provides numerous kinds of safety-related data, including patient data, health records, calculated risk levels, suggested medications, graphical illustrations, graphs and trees, and others. These features help clinicians in that they can compare after and before situations to determine the result of various treatments.

Besides the automatic processes, the interactions between healthcare providers and patients are incorporated into the system through interfaces. This integration also helps to facilitate how medical data originating from diagnostic sensors, machine learning predictive models, doctors, and patients are transformed into useful information. As a result, the CDSS supplies a more effective instrument of decision-making in managing a patient's present condition relative to his or her medical history. Finally, CDSS fosters a data-inspired, patient-centered model of healthcare to improve the efficiency and effectiveness of working clinical decisions.

### 10.1.2 Evolution of CDSS

The development of CDSS is marked by various technological milestones, all contributing to the enhancement of its capabilities. The early CDSS were rule-based systems, which mainly used the curated knowledge basis and if-then logic. These systems, such as MYCIN, were designed in the early 1970s for detecting infectious diseases and demonstrated the progress of CDSS systems to improve the decision-making aspect. The only drawback that was associated with that system was the fact that it relied on knowledge bases, which were static and therefore had limited room for adaptability and scalability. Particularly when the volume and the complexity of the medical data boomed exponentially, these systems usually failed. Now the advent of artificial intelligence (AI), as well as the usage of machine learning (ML), has transformed these knowledge bases from static, rule-based systems to dynamic, data-driven platforms (Sutton, 2020). Modern systems are able to make use of these advanced algorithms to be able to identify as well as learn intricate patterns from the data, which allows them to present their predictions in a probabilistic manner rather than being deterministic in their recommendations. This transition from static to fixed to dynamic has made the CDSS systems more precise while improving their adaptable use in real-world problems, as depicted in Figure 10.2. A classic example is AI systems, which can find patterns in image data and assist practitioners in identifying diseases such as cancer and other neurodegenerative diseases.

Moving to unstructured data, the CDSS has been using natural language processing (NLP) to interpret clinical notes, research articles, and patient

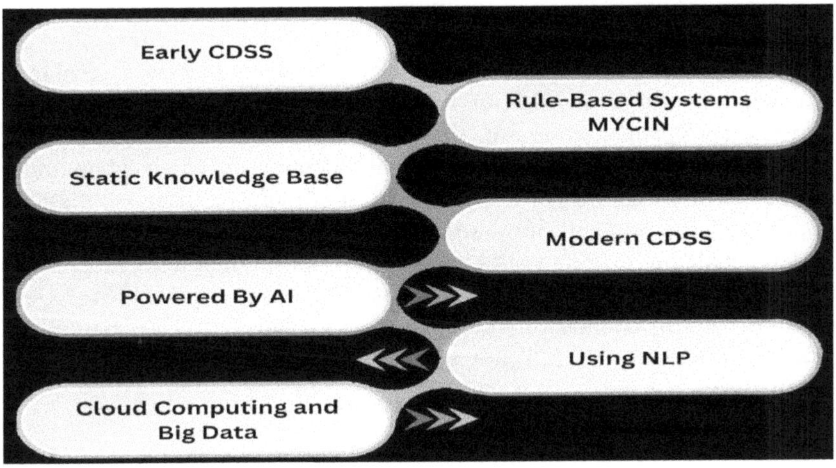


*Figure 10.2* Evolution of CDSSs

feedback to broaden its sphere. The NLP algorithms can identify the information available in these sources and make it available to the systems, thus increasing their ability to make decisions using appropriate contextual information. This capability is most helpful regarding information, which is always overwhelming to clinicians facing an expanding body of knowledge about medicine. The five main concepts considered as the basis of the development of CDSS systems have also incorporated cloud computing and big data analytics into this area. These would help the system aggregate and analyze large datasets from multiple sources while not worrying about the system's scale, thus making the system more resilient (Berner, 2016). Due to these technologies, CDSS can operate in real time since it pulls data for the individual from EHRs, wearable devices, and genomics to meet their bizarre requirements and recommend interventions based on their environment and lifestyle. The transformation of the paradigm from the rule-based to the AI approaches or the AI application, specifically in healthcare 4.0, has enhanced the development of CDSS. However, this implementation has some adverse effects, which include explainability and trust. The traditional systems were more transparent in terms of providing reasoning for their recommendations, on the other hand, the AI systems usually function as black boxes, making it difficult for practitioners to understand the rationale behind certain decisions. The nature of AI systems makes this issue a pressing one to be addressed for the adoption as well as the efficacy of CDSS in clinical practices.

Therefore, this chapter aims to provide a comprehensive survey of how CDSS performs, with a focus on the implementation of AI to enhance its capabilities. The chapter explores its evolution, application and challenges of CDSS as well as contributes to the growing body of knowledge at the intersection of healthcare and technology. Another objective that has been a part of this chapter is to elucidate how AI has helped to address the challenges that traditional systems face, as well as how it makes the system more accurate in terms of decision-making. The chapter also aligns in exploring various implementations of AI, which include machine learning, deep learning, and NLP, concerning CDSS. The chapter is also focused on understanding various challenges that are associated with the usage of CDSS in modern aspects. Some of the challenges that are prevalent in the context of modern medicine include issues relating to data quality, algorithmic bias, and the black-box nature of AI. Addressing of these issues is paramount, and therefore the chapter provides insights to seek the development of better CDSS solutions, which follow such guidelines.

## 10.2 LITERATURE REVIEW

The initial aspect of the development of CDSS was the introduction of rule-based systems, a popular example of the same being MYCIN, which makes use of heuristic rules to provide recommendations based on if-then rules (Topol, 2019). These systems were considered ahead of their time in helping medical diagnosis but had their limitations, which included but were not limited to the aspect of more complex data, high-dimensional datasets, and more dynamic patient conditions. Therefore, it is seen that the usage of AI marked itself a paradigm shift in the functioning of CDSS, helping them to cater to vast datasets and also understand patterns that were not discernible in the past. ML as technology has also helped further the advancement of CDSS with its implementation of various techniques like logistic regression, decision trees, and support vector machine. As early as 2016, Obermeyer and Emanuel (2016) implemented the usage of ML as an aspect to determine hospital readmission. They highlighted that the ML-based systems were able to improve patient outcomes efficiently while also reducing the aspects of healthcare costs for the people. The integration of ensemble methods, in this regard, has also been explored in terms of enhancing the accuracy as well as efficiency of the system by the usage of multiple algorithms being aggregated (Chen & Guestrin, 2016; Li, 2020). Furthering the scope of CDSS, even deep learning was implemented to handle the complexity of growing data (Mandel et al., 2016). The usage of medical images as well as the analysis of the same was only handled by the usage of better developed neural networks. Their efficacy in detecting diseases has been evident through many studies, with Esteva et al. (2017) highlighting the potential that deep learning has in terms of achieving dermatologist-level accuracy in diagnosing skin cancer. Successful implementations of context and time-based algorithms like recurrent neural networks (RNNs) and long short-term memory (LSTM), by Lipton (2015), show promise in the field of medical analysis furthered with AI and deep learning. It must also be pointed out that even natural language processing (NLP) has been a part of the development of medical AI, with successful implementations showing how unstructured data is being used. Other known models such as BERT and GPT can already handle the clinical datasets for the medical side of NLP. The effectiveness of the same has been demonstrated by Lee et al. (2020), who showed how a large language model (LLM) trained in medical data can understand the context of doctor notes and thereby help in making appropriate predictions for the same (Lundberg, 2017). Such a capability of AI helps to automate tasks such as cohort identification and adverse event prediction, which rely heavily on textual data.

CDSS has been evolved by applying a rule-based approach in developing MYCIN in 1970 to recent developments in deep learning like LLM. Table 10.1 has information regarding CDSS focusing on different disease diagnostics and treatment coming up over the years.

## 10.3 INTEGRATION WITH HEALTHCARE WORKFLOWS

To make the AI-based CDSS system effective as well as efficient, it is important to have seamless integration into the healthcare workflow. Therefore, to highlight the process of the same, this section explores the strategies of integration into the CDSS systems. The very first step in the deployment strategy is often to include the CDSS system in the EHR systems. This integration would allow the AI models to be able to get context-aware data, which helps them to make better recommendations in line with the patient encounters and medical information. This kind of integration would also ensure that there is real-time support from the system and the insights are available from the start of the care treatment, streamlining the decision-making process. The integration of CDSS also calls for the development of sophisticated data centers that can store such vast amounts of data as well as relay the same to the models for better predictive capabilities. A critical application of this integrated CDSS system is the aspect of personalized medicines. The presence of patient-specific data allows for the models to tailor treatment strategies which are only effective for the specific genome of the patient and thereby increase healing chances. The AI models that are trained on large data sets can identify the genetic, environmental, and lifestyle factors, which progress the disease and suggest corrective measures in the form of medicines that cater to the patient only under consideration. For instance, AI-driven pharmacogenomic tools analyze genetic variations to predict drug efficacy and adverse reactions, enabling precision in medication prescribing.

*Table 10.1* Some CDSSs developed and published over the last three decades

| *CDSS name* | *Year introduced* | *Primary focus* | *Key features* |
|---|---|---|---|
| MYCIN (Shortliffe, 1976) | 1970s | Antibiotic selection for bacterial infections | Rule-based expert system, used backward chaining, focused on treating infections like sepsis and meningitis. |
| Iliad (Warner et al., 1985) | 1980s | Diagnostic support | Probabilistic reasoning using Bayesian networks, supported differential diagnosis across specialties. |
| DXplain (Barnett et al., 1987) | 1987 | Diagnostic support | Provided ranked differential diagnoses based on symptoms, diseases, and patient history. |
| Arden Syntax (Hripcsak et al., 1990) | 1990 | Standardization of CDSS rules | Developed a standard language for writing and sharing medical logic modules (MLMs) for CDS. |
| Oncology Expert Advisor (Shortliffe & Perreault, 2001) | 1990s | Oncology treatment planning | AI-based system for personalized cancer treatment, using historical data and expert input. |
| MedLEE (Friedman et al., 1998) | 1990s | NLP for medicine | Extracted structured clinical data from unstructured text like medical notes, enabling automated analysis. |
| ISABEL (Ramnarayan et al., 2008) | 2000 | Pediatric and general diagnostic support | Suggested diagnoses based on symptoms entered into its web-based interface; widely adopted for its intuitive design. |
| OpenCDS (Kawamoto & Lobach, 2007) | 2010 | Open-source CDS framework | Enabled integration of standards-based CDS into EHR systems, supporting large-scale deployment of evidence-based guidelines. |
| Sepsis CDS Tools (Henry et al., 2015) | 2010s | Early sepsis detection | Real-time analytics to detect and alert clinicians about sepsis using predictive models integrated with hospital EHRs. |
| Infermedica (Chmielewski et al., 2016) | 2012 | Symptom checker and triage | AI-powered diagnostic engine used for patient triage in telemedicine and healthcare apps, utilized knowledge graphs for reasoning. |
| Watson for Oncology (IBM Watson Health, 2016) | 2014 | Oncology treatment recommendations | AI-based CDS by IBM, processed medical literature, and suggested treatments for cancer patients, considering clinical guidelines. |

(*Continued*)

*Table 10.1* (Continued) Some CDSSs developed and published over the last three decades

| *CDSS name* | *Year introduced* | *Primary focus* | *Key features* |
|---|---|---|---|
| DeepMind's Streams (Moor et al., 2019) | 2016 | Acute kidney injury (AKI) detection | AI-powered mobile app that alerted clinicians to signs of AKI based on patient data, designed in collaboration with NHS hospitals. |
| PathAI (Steiner et al., 2018) | 2016 | Pathology diagnosis | Machine learning-based system for improving accuracy in pathology diagnoses, focusing on cancers like breast and prostate. |
| Buoy Health (Buoy Health, 2017) | 2017 | Symptom checker and health navigation | AI-powered system for patient self-triage, guiding users to appropriate care resources based on symptoms and context. |
| Viz.ai (Viz.ai, 2018) | 2018 | Stroke detection | AI-driven system for detecting large vessel occlusions (LVO) in stroke patients from CT scans, sending alerts to specialists in real time. |
| Dreem CDS (Arnal et al., 2020) | 2021 | Sleep medicine | AI-driven system for analyzing sleep patterns, used in diagnosing sleep disorders and improving treatment plans. |
| Biofourmis Biovitals (Steinhubl et al., 2019) | 2021 | Remote patient monitoring | AI platform analyzing continuous data from wearable devices to predict patient deterioration and support early intervention. |
| Google Health Derm Assist (Google Health, 2021) | 2021 | Dermatology | AI-powered tool for skin condition identification, guiding patients and physicians to appropriate care for dermatological issues. |
| Qure.ai (Quare.a i, 2022) | 2022 | Radiology AI | AI-based system for interpreting medical imaging, including chest X-rays and head CTs, used in resource-limited settings to augment diagnostic capacity. |
| Healthie.AI (Healthie.AI, 2022) | 2022 | Comprehensive EHR-integrated CDS | Provided predictive analytics, alerts, and care recommendations, integrating seamlessly with EHRs for primary and specialty care. |

It must be highlighted that an integrated CDSS system not only is beneficial for patients in terms of personalized care but also helps in the optimization of healthcare systems and resources in the medical fraternity. The protective analytics model when integrated with hospital management systems can cater not only to patient outcomes but also to patient admissions, thereby helping the hospital to manage its resources proactively. With a prior alert of upcoming patient admissions, the hospital will be able to plan for its staff and resource needs, as well as priority payments, which are based on the severity of their diseases. Such an optimized workflow allows the hospital to ensure timely care delivery as well as manage its resources without burdening its caregivers. It can be noted that an important feature of CDSS system implementation is the communication capability of the existing clinical systems. These integrated systems must be capable of contacting the pre-existing clinical systems in a manner that is observable and comprehensible. There is a need to implement standards like HL7 (Health Level Seven) and FHIR (Fast Healthcare Interoperability Resources) that enable the information exchange between such systems. Such standards would enable harmonized integration between the CDSS tools and the healthcare ecosystem without compromising on the data, exchange, and personal information recording aspects of the healthcare services, with an aspect that is optimal for healthcare services.

## 10.4 CONCLUSION

Integrating AI in clinical decision support systems (CDSSs) is one of the most revolutionary advancements in contemporary healthcare. Since the application of machine learning, deep learning, and natural language processing, AI-based CDSS improves diagnostic performance, individualizes the treatment, and optimizes the practice of clinicians. This survey has described the transition from engineering-rule-based systems to black-box complex AI models to understand that such systems can process different and intricate healthcare information resources, from imaging and EHRs to genomics. Nevertheless, the application of AI in CDSS is facing several challenges. This is a considerable challenge to data scientists who continue to grapple with other challenges, such as data quality, interpretability, and algorithm bias. Since precision medicine is gradually becoming the focus in healthcare delivery, AI's role in developing CDSS is seen as strategic to the realization of precision medicine in the future. However, for the broader implementation to be successful, the work needs to collaborate with other fields to guarantee that the systems in question are explainable, interpretable, and scalable within various clinical practices. By effectively overcoming these challenges, AI-CDSS will be optimized to achieve optimal benefits and change healthcare globally.

## REFERENCES


Arnal, P. J., et al. (2020). The Dreem headband: Validation of an EEG-based sleep-monitoring device for clinical trials. *Journal of Sleep Research*, *29*(1), e12920.

Barnett, G. O., Cimino, J. J., Hupp, J. A., & Hoffer, E. P. (1987). DXplain: An evolving diagnostic decision-support system. *JAMA*, *258*(1), 67–74.

Beeler, P. E., Bates, D. W., & Hug, B. L. (2014). Clinical decision support systems. *Swiss Medical Weekly*, *144*, w14073.

Berner, E. S., & La Lande, T. J. (2016). Overview of clinical decision support systems. In *Clinical decision support systems: Theory and practice* (pp. 1–17). Springer International Publishing.

Buoy Health, Inc. (2017). *Buoy health symptom checker.* [Online]. Available: https://www.buoyhealth.com.

Chen, T., & Guestrin, C. (2016, August). Xgboost: A scalable tree boosting system. In *Proceedings of the 22nd acm sigkdd international conference on knowledge discovery and data mining* (KDD '16) (pp. 785–794). Association for Computing Machinery. https://doi.org/10.1145/2939672.2939785.

Chmielewski, M., & Borowczyk, M. (2016). *A framework for building explainable AI solutions for medical diagnosis.* Proceedings of the 2016 Federated Conference on Computer Science and Information Systems (pp. 1439–1442).

Esteva, A., Kuprel, B., Novoa, R. A., Ko, J., Swetter, S. M., Blau, H. M., & Thrun, S. (2017). Dermatologist-level classification of skin cancer with deep neural networks. *Nature*, *542*(7639), 115–118.

Friedman, C., & Hripcsak, G. (1998). Natural language processing and its future in medicine. *Academic Medicine*, *73*(8), 890–895.

Google Health. (2021). *Derm assist: Helping people identify skin conditions.* [Online]. Available: https://health.google/derm-assist.

Healthie.AI. (2022). *Next-generation clinical decision support for EHR integration.* [Online]. Available: https://healthie.ai

Henry, K. E., & Hager, D. N. (2015). A targeted real-time early warning score (TREWScore) for septic shock. *Science Translational Medicine*, *7*(299), 299ra122.

Hripcsak, G., & Wigertz, O. B. (1990). *Arden syntax for medical logic modules.* Proceedings of the Annual Symposium on Computer Application in Medical Care, pp. 200–204.

IBM Watson Health. (2016). *Watson for oncology: Advancing cancer care.* [Online]. Available: https://www.ibm.com/watson-health/oncology

Kawamoto, K., & Lobach, D. F. (2007). Proposal for Fulfilling Strategic Objectives of the U.S. Roadmap for National Action on Decision Support through a Service-oriented Architecture Leveraging HL7 Services. *Journal of the American Medical Informatics Association*, *14*(2), 146–155.

Lee, J., Yoon, W., Kim, S., Kim, D., Kim, S., So, C. H., & Kang, J. (2020). BioBERT: a pre-trained biomedical language representation model for biomedical text mining. *Bioinformatics*, *36*(4), 1234–1240.

Li, T., Sahu, A. K., Talwalkar, A., & Smith, V. (2020). Federated learning: Challenges, methods, and future directions. *IEEE Signal Processing Magazine*, *37*(3), 50–60.

Lipton, Z. C. (2015). Learning to diagnose with LSTM recurrent neural networks. *arXiv preprint arXiv:1511.03677.*

Lundberg, S. (2017). A unified approach to interpreting model predictions. *arXiv preprint arXiv:1705.07874.*

Mandel, J. C., Kreda, D. A., Mandl, K. D., Kohane, I. S., & Ramoni, R. B. (2016). SMART on FHIR: A standards-based, interoperable apps platform for electronic health records. *Journal of the American Medical Informatics Association, 23*(5), 899–908.

Moor, M., & Claassen, J. (2019). *Early recognition of sepsis with Gaussian process temporal convolutional networks and dynamic time warping.* Proceedings of the 4th Machine Learning for Healthcare Conference (pp. 2–26).

Musen, M. A., Middleton, B., & Greenes, R. A. (2021). Clinical decision-support systems. In *Biomedical informatics: Computer applications in health care and biomedicine* (pp. 795–840). Springer International Publishing.

Obermeyer, Z., & Emanuel, E. J. (2016). Predicting the future—big data, machine learning, and clinical medicine. *New England Journal of Medicine, 375*(13), 1216–1219.

Qure.ai. (2022). *AI solutions for radiology.* [Online]. Available: https://qure.ai.

Ramnarayan, P., & Cronje, N. (2008). ISABEL: A web-based differential diagnostic aid for pediatrics: results from an initial performance evaluation. *Archives of Disease in Childhood, 93*(8), 633–635.

Shortliffe, E. H. (1976). *Computer-based medical consultations: MYCIN.* Elsevier.

Shortliffe, E. H., & Perreault, L. E. (2001). *Medical informatics: Computer applications in health care and biomedicine.* Springer.

Steiner, D. F., & Chen, P. H. (2018). Impact of deep learning assistance on the histopathologic review of lymph nodes for metastatic breast cancer. *American Journal of Surgical Pathology, 42*(12), 1636–1646.

Steinhubl, S. R., et al. (2019). Remote monitoring and wearable devices in health care. *Nature Biotechnology, 37*, 429–436.

Sutton, R. T., Pincock, D., Baumgart, D. C., Sadowski, D. C., Fedorak, R. N., & Kroeker, K. I. (2020). An overview of clinical decision support systems: Benefits, risks, and strategies for success. *NPJ Digital Medicine, 3*(1), 17.

Topol, E. J. (2019). High-performance medicine: the convergence of human and artificial intelligence. *Nature Medicine, 25*(1), 44–56.

Viz.ai, Inc. (2018). *Viz LVO: AI-powered stroke detection.* [Online]. Available: https://www.viz.ai.

Warner, H. R., Olmsted, C. M., & Rutherford, B. D. (1985). HELP—a program for medical decision-making. *Computers and Biomedical Research, 18*(5), 377–395.

# Index

1956 Dartmouth Conference, 26

American Cancer Society, 118
American Medical Association (AMA), 38
Antimicrobial resistance (AMR), 51, 56–59
Artificial intelligence (AI), 6, 8–9, 81–82
  advantages, 39–40
  challenges, 16–20
  computational analysis, 37–38
  domain of, 83–85
  drug development complexities, 32–33
  drug discovery, 33–34
  features of, 10
  future scope of, 20–21
  health diagnosis, 35–36
  history of, 83
  medical applications, 38–39
  precision medicine, 34–35
  roles and capabilities, 40–42
Artificial intelligence in medicine (AIM), 118
Artificial neural networks (ANNs), 13, 30, 69, 72, 81, 117, 125, 172
Assisted reproductive technology (ART), 93

Basic Local Alignment Search Tool (BLAST), 153
Bio-psycho-social, 16
Biomedical science, 5–6
  key aspects of, 7
Biometric monitoring devices (BMDs), 174
Biopsies, 102
BIOSTATARTM system, 132
Boosting techniques, 123

Cardiac assist device (CAD), 38, 106, 118, 133, 134
Cardiotocography (CTG), 81, 86
Chemotherapy, 130, 138
Classification and regression trees (CARTs), 91, 104
Clinical decision support systems (CDSSs), 188–190
  application of, 196
  evolution of, 190–192
  healthcare workflows, 193–196
  literature review, 192–193
Closed-loop control system, 132–135
CloudUPDRS, 39
Clustered Regularly Interspaced Short Palindromic Repeats (CRISPR), 5, 155
Colorectal cancer, 101, 104, 108
Comprehensive blood glycopeptide spectra analysis (CSGSA), 92
Computer-aided fetal evaluations (CAFEs), 81
Computer-assisted detection or diagnosis (CAD), 104, 106
Continuous glucose monitoring (CGM), 69, 71–73, 76
Control systems, 116, 133, 138
Convolutional neural networks (CNNs), 29, 30, 36, 52, 70, 72, 74, 75, 84, 154, 159
Copy number variations (CNVs), 87
Coronary computed tomographic angiography (CCTA), 38

COVID-19, 5, 29, 31–32, 37, 52, 55, 57, 61, 62, 171

Decision trees (DTs), 30, 69, 71, 75, 85, 104, 123–124, 192
Deep learning (DL)
  abstract layers, 121–123
  cardiac disease detection, 29
  cervical cancer, 86–88
  Chromputer, 154
  clinical decision support systems, 188–196
  colposcopy, 88
  convolutional neural networks, 75
  diabetes, 30–31
  diabetes management, 71–73
  diabetic risk prediction, 69
  diagnostic imaging, 52, 54
  disease progression prediction, 171
  domain of AI, 83–85
  drug discovery, 13, 15, 56
  emergence of, 26
  endometrial cancer, 89
  epidemiology, 60
  functional genomics, 155
  gastroesophageal reflux, 106
  infectious disease diagnosis, 52
  machine learning, 174–176
  medical imaging, 36
  ovarian cancer, 91
  structural genomics, 156
Deep neural networks (DNNs), 31, 32, 159, 172
DeepConvNet, 75
Diabetes mellitus (DM), 67–69
  AI-enabled diagnostics, 70–71
  challenges, 77–78
  continuous glucose monitoring, 76
  diabetic foot ulcers, 75–76
  diabetic retinopathy, 74–75
  ethical considerations, 77–78
  management techniques, 71–73
  personalized treatment, 73–74
  preventive management, 76
  remote, 77
  risk prediction, 69–70
Diabetic foot ulcers (DFUs), 75, 76
Diabetic retinopathy (DR), 36, 68–72, 74–75, 78
Diagnosis of diseases, 28–29
  COVID-19, 31–32
  diabetes, 30–31
  heart diseases, 29
Distant metastasis rates (DMR), 88–89
Drug delivery strategies, 116–117, 127
  biological systems
    cancer treatments, 138–139
    cardiac ailments, 133–135
    gastrointestinal system, 135–138
    insulin delivery, 131–133
  development, 139
  fundamentals of
    categories of, 120–123
    growing role of, 117–119
    medicine and pharmaceutical industry, 119–120
  machine learning models
    artificial neural networks, 125
    Boost, 123
    decision trees, 123–124
    feedback system control, 126
    k-nearest neighbors, 124–125
    logistic regression, 125
    Naïve Bayes, 126
    random forest, 123–124
    set covering machine, 126
    support vector machine, 124
  nanotechnology, 126–129
    nanomedicine, 129–131
    nanorobots, 131
Drug–target interactions, 128

Electrocardiogram (EKG), 39
Electronic health record (EHR) systems, 11, 18, 35, 39, 40, 60, 67, 69, 71, 74, 76, 77, 117, 158, 171, 179, 188
Endoscopy, 100, 101, 106, 112, 118, 135, 137
Enhanced Detection System for Healthcare-Associated Transmission (EDS-HAT), 158
Enterion capsule, 135
Epithelial ovarian cancer (EOC), 92
Expert system, 26, 83, 153, 167, 172
Extensively drug-resistant (XDR), 57

Federation of Gynecology and Obstetrics (FIGO), 89
Feedback system control (FSC), 126
Fractional flow reverse computed tomography (FFRCT), 38
Free-energy minimization, 34
Fuzzy logic control (FLC), 133, 134

Gallstones, 101
Gastric intestinal metaplasia (GIM), 99
Gastroenterology, 100
 anatomy and function, 100–101
 artificial intelligence, 102–103
  challenges, 111–112
  diagnostics, 105–106
  prevention, 103–104
  prognosis, 108–109, 111
  treatment, 106–108
 common conditions, 101
 diagnostic tools, 101–102
 research and techniques, 102
 treatment modalities, 102
Gastroesophageal reflux disease (GERD), 101, 108
Gastrointestinal inflammation disorders (GID), 101
Gaussian interaction, 124, 128
General Data Protection Regulation (GDPR), 77
Genomics
 applications of
  comparative, 154–155
  functional, 155
  structural, 156
 chronological order of, 153–154
 epigenomics, 156–157
 ethical aspects of, 160–161
 healthcare professionals, 158–160
 human genome project, 152
 impact of, 160
 limitations of, 160
 metagenomics, 157–158
Geographic Information Systems (GIS), 61
Gluten sensitivity disorder, 101
Google DeepMind, 27, 118
Graph Information Bottleneck (GIB), 108
Gynecology
 clinical advantage of AI, 86
  cervical cancer, 86–89
  cervical intraepithelial neoplasia, 86–89
  endometrial cancer, 89–91
  ovarian cancer, 91–93

Health Insurance Portability and Accountability Act (HIPAA), 77, 111
Healthcare research, 3–5, 9, 11
 applications of, 9
  drug discovery, 13, 15
  medical imaging and diagnostics, 10–14
  mental health support, 15–18
Hepatitis, 56, 57, 101
Hepatology, 100
Hidden Markov models (HMMs), 153
HPV testing, 86–88
Human leukocyte antigen-DR (HLA-DR), 32
Hyperglycemia (type 1 diabetes), 67, 131

IBM Watson, 27, 74, 176
In vitro fertilization (IVF), 81, 84
Infectious diseases, 51–52
 antimicrobial resistance, 58–59
 application of, 63–64
 challenges, 62–63
 diagnosis, 52
  imaging, 52, 54
  microbial identification, 54
  point-of-care, 54–55
  predictive and risk assessment, 55–56
  syndromic, 55
 epidemiology, 60
 ethical considerations, 62–63
 outbreak prediction, 60–62
 surveillance and global health, 59–60
 treatment, 56
  drug discovery, 56–57
  optimization, 57–58
  personalized medicine, 58
Intel Capital, 118
InteliSite, 135
IntelliCap, 135, 136
International Diabetes Federation (IDF), 67
Irritable bowel syndrome (IBS), 101, 137

K-nearest neighbors (KNNs), 30, 92, 124–125

Least squares regularization, 128
Logistic regression (LR), 125, 172, 192

Machine learning (ML), 8, 13, 26, 28–30, 32–34, 51–52, 55–57, 59–61, 63, 64, 69, 72–75, 83–85, 92, 93, 103, 106, 120–129, 150, 157–159, 174, 190; *see also* Deep learning

Machine learning-based disease diagnoses (MLBD), 29
Magnetic resonance imaging (MRI), 88–90, 169
MARIA framework, 31
Mazor Robotics, 121
Mean arterial blood pressure (MABP), 134, 135
Medical Device Regulation (MDR), 19
Medical imaging
  applications, 36–37
Medical sciences, 167
  adoption, 179
  challenges, 177–178, 181–182
  disease progression prediction, 171–172
  drug design, 172–173
  growth acceleration, 172–173
  healthcare systems, 168–169
  machine learning, 174–176
  medical imaging interpretation, 169
  opportunities of, 176–177
  recommodations, 180–181
  remote monitoring, 173–174
  risks, 178–179
Mesoporous silica nanoparticles (MSNPs), 129
Microchip, 116, 131
Microsatellite instability (MSI) tests, 90, 108
Model Expert System (MES), 172
Model predictive control (MPC), 133, 134
Multidrug-resistant (MDR), 57
MYCIN, 153, 167, 190, 192, 193

Naïve Bayes (NB), 30, 126
National Institutes of Health (NIH), 118
Natural language processing (NLP), 8, 26, 51, 54, 69, 71, 77, 117, 122, 150, 154, 190, 193, 196
Neurofuzzy integrated system, 29
Next-generation sequencing (NGS), 54, 87, 90, 152, 159
NVIDIA, 159

Pancreatic ductal adenocarcinoma (PDAC), 129
Pancreatitis, 101
Pap smear, 86–88
Pathologists, 169
Peptic ulcers, 101
Polymerase chain reaction (PCR), 52
Predicting Response to Depression Treatment (PReDicT), 176–177

Quantitative structure–activity relationship (QSAR), 34

Radio frequency identification (RFID), 174
Radiologists, 10, 54, 88, 90, 91, 93, 169
Random forests (RFs), 30, 71, 123–124, 172
Recurrent neural networks (RNNs), 71, 72, 76, 192
Reinforcement learning (RL), 8, 71–73, 84, 85, 134, 150
Remote patient monitoring (RPM), 173

Set covering machine (SCM), 126
Severe cute respiratory syndrome coronavirus 2 (SARS-CoV-2), 32, 158
Silica nanoparticle (SNP), 134
Silicasomes, 129
Single-nucleotide polymorphisms (SNPs), 73, 155
Sliding Mode Control (SMC), 133
Software as a medical device (SaMD), 38
Software in medical devices (SiMD), 38
Speech technology, 123
Stool tests, 102
Supervised learning, 8, 31, 71, 72, 84, 85, 99, 122, 128
Support vector machines (SVMs), 30, 34, 69, 71, 75, 124, 158, 172

Three-dimensional (3D) printing technology, 33, 86

Ulcerative Colitis (UC), 101, 110
Ultrasound, 91, 93, 100, 101, 116, 161, 172
Unsupervised learning, 8, 71, 72, 84, 85, 99, 122
Up-conversion core/porous silica shell nanotheranostics (UCSNs), 130

World Health Organization (WHO), 30, 86

For Product Safety Concerns and Information please contact our EU
representative GPSR@taylorandfrancis.com
Taylor & Francis Verlag GmbH, Kaufingerstraße 24, 80331 München, Germany

www.ingramcontent.com/pod-product-compliance
Ingram Content Group UK Ltd.
Pitfield, Milton Keynes, MK11 3LW, UK
UKHW020202200926
475702UK00004B/573

* 9 7 8 1 0 3 2 8 6 5 7 4 4 *